Directions: Clarity For Medical Group Leaders

Mark F. Weiss

Published by The Mark F. Weiss Law Firm, a Professional Corporation

1227 De La Vina Street

Santa Barbara, CA 93101

310-843-2800

For information about Mark F. Weiss's services and speaking, please call 310-843-2800 or email request@advisorylawgroup.com. Free articles, videos, podcasts and the archive of the Advisory e-Alert, our electronic newsletter, are available at www.advisorylawgroup.com.

Visit www.advisorylawgroup.com to subscribe to our complimentary monthly e-Alert and to follow the link to Mark's frequently updated Wisdom. Applied. blog.

INTRODUCTION

Changing Your Thinking.

Joseph Schumpter, the Austrian-born economist and sociologist who spent most of his career teaching at Harvard University, posited that capitalism is by nature a method of economic change and not only never is, but never can be stationary.

Schumpeter used the term "creative destruction" to describe incessant change from within. He saw it as the essential fact about capitalism. In his words, "it is what capitalism consists in and what every capitalist concern has got to live in."

Healthcare is changing – a prime example of Schumpeter's theory of creative destruction.

The problem is that many leaders of physician groups as well as many entrepreneurial
physicians don't fully understand what the problem is.

How can you find a solution, how can you engage in the right development of strategy, and how can you to plan your, or your group's, future unless you have some tools to help clarify your thinking?

This short book contains a collection of thoughts as thinking tools. Each one is intended to instruct, inform, and even more so, cause you to give pause to instruct and inform yourself.

Enjoy!

Mark F. Weiss

CONTENTS

INTRODUCTION

Changing Your Thinking.

Joseph Schumpter, the Austrian-born economist and sociologist who spent most of his career teaching at Harvard University, posited that capitalism is by nature a method of economic change and not only never is, but never can be stationary.

Schumpeter used the term "creative destruction" to describe incessant change from within. He saw it as the essential fact about capitalism. In his words, "it is what capitalism consists in and what every capitalist concern has got to live in."

Healthcare is changing – a prime example of Schumpeter's theory of creative destruction.

The problem is that many leaders of physician groups as well as many entrepreneurial physicians don't fully understand what the problem is.

How can you find a solution, how can you engage in the right development of strategy, and how can you to plan your, or your group's, future unless you have some tools to help clarify your thinking?

This short book contains a collection of thoughts as thinking tools. Each one is intended to instruct, inform, and even more so, cause you to give pause to instruct and inform yourself.

Enjoy!

Mark F. Weiss

Strategy

THE MAGIC HAT AND MEDICAL GROUP STRATEGY

When my son, Noah, was little, he told me that he had a magic hat. When he wore it, he could see the future.

Most medical group leaders could use a hat like that. Not that it's really needed. In many cases the writing on the wall is clear.

Hospitals are building monopolies, employing and otherwise "aligning" physicians. National groups are competing as if on steroids. And many local medical groups feel as if they're sailing in a thimble facing down a battleship.

So what's your strategy? I hope it's not to float with the tide. That's almost everyone else's strategy.

Oh, you're wearing your magic hat.

MARRIAGE AND MEDICAL GROUP MERGERS

Medical group mergers are a lot like marriages.

Some are actual mergers. The formerly separate groups really do become one. For richer, for poorer, in sickness and in health. So if one of the merged practice sites closes, the partners based there are reassigned. There's still love, or as much as there can be in a merger as opposed to an actual marriage.

But too common these days are mergers that are simply temporal, for market share, for beefing up for a private equity deal, or to share contract rates. These are a bit like marriages for the purpose of obtaining a green card. So if merged-in group "A" loses its exclusive contract or if providing services at that site no longer makes economic sense to the group as a whole, then everyone in "A," from partners to part-timers are shown the door.

The ties that bind versus the lies that say goodbye.

Sure, unlike immigration love, less than heartfelt medical group merger isn't a federal crime. If you're in control of the merger, "do it until it no longer feels good" may be exactly what you're looking for.

But if your group is the merger target, make sure you know what kind of marriage your intended has in mind.

THREE STRATEGIC LESSONS FOR INDEPENDENT MEDICAL GROUPS

As healthcare entities become larger they appear as formidable competitors in the marketplace.

So what's an independent group to do?

November 25, 1863. The Civil War. The Battle of Missionary Ridge outside of Chattanooga.

For several months, the Confederate Army held Union forces at bay within a tight semicircular defensive position. Then the Union Army under General Grant launched a coordinated attack against both sides of the Confederate line as well as at its center. The side attacks had little success. But at the middle, the Union troops breached the line and then . . . things seemingly fell apart for all. Both sides issued confusing orders to their troops: What were the objectives? What was to be defended? But the outcome was the collapse of the Confederate defense.

The first lesson: Seemingly strong competitors have a weak point and their large size makes them overly fragile. Find the point of weakness and exploit it. Grant sent his forces to attack at three points. Only one attack out of three hit a weak point, but that was enough.

The second lesson. A large competitor cannot deal with the confusion quickly enough to save itself. They are too organized, too centralized, too stiff. Although both the Union and the Confederate troops fighting at the center received confusing orders, the Union troops were better at observing the situation and at taking advantage of it. (An illustration of Boyd's OODA loop: Observe – Orient – Decide – Act.

The third lesson? The first two are so important for you to consider that the third will only get in the way.

HEDGE OR HEDGEHOG OR ???

The initial notion of a hedge fund was that its investment risk was reduced through a "hedge," an off-setting investment.

I've noticed that many medical practices, from small office based groups, to large hospital-based groups, and even to national groups, hedge, too.

But that hedge tends to fall into two distinct classes: Acting like a hedgehog and acting out hedges.

Those in the hedgehog class are insular, perhaps protecting their turf but doing nothing to expand it.

Of course, "turf" is capable of different definitions. For example, for an office-based practice it might be relying on historic referral patterns. For a large hospital-based group it might be relying on an exclusive contract with a single hospital. And, for a regional single-specialty group it might be relying on the survivability of the single specialty model.

Those who are hedging view the world differently. Rather than simply building an insular hedge around their business, they expand outside of that hedge, taking on other business, in some ways both related and unrelated.

What is really interesting, and what many, if not all, have ever considered, is the possibility of being both. Perhaps the real issue is not being big or of being small, or of being a hedgehog or a hedger, but instead being all of those things at once.

MERGER: FALLEN FROM GRACE

Grace, not her real name, was very pretty. Long blonde hair. Tall. Fun.

But we used to joke that she could never develop a relationship because she didn't like her suitors' financial statements.

It's not that financial considerations don't enter into the larger issue of finding a desirable spouse. It's that they're only one slice of what is important.

Medical group mergers aren't much different.

Mating two weakly performing groups rarely yields a successful future. And, a poorly performing group can be an anchor, dragging down a previously thriving practice.

But even two balance sheet appropriate candidates can be the match made in hell.

Group culture, governance styles, and what I call the jerk-to-normal ratio, among other soft factors, are often more important than tallying the ability to put cash in the bank.

As to Grace, that's another story.

ALTERNATIVE TO COMMODITIZED PRACTICE

As the chill of Obamacare becomes felt, more and more physicians are looking for alternatives to commoditized medical practice.

For example, practice alternatives include concierge medicine, mobile practice, franchise operations, and what I term "disruptive medicine" – the creation of either, or both, new technologies and new delivery systems.

Within the four walls of what is now viewed as traditional medical practice, physicians are generally placed, and have placed themselves, into silo-like specialties. In some cases, specialists within one specialty complain that those from another are "poaching" their territory — take imaging studies being done by cardiologists, for example, and the reaction that engenders among radiologists.

On the other hand, many of the ways out require that physicians see themselves in roles larger than a single specialty or see the walls of their specialty as subject to a retrofit. Take, for example, the cardiologists in the above example.

So, allow me to knock down some walls and really mix metaphors: If you're on a ship that you know is sinking, and sinking fast, you can take the lifeboat, or swim for safety. You can also stay on board and cry about your "fate." You do have a choice.

HOW MEDICAL GROUPS GET MIRED FIGHTING THE LAST WAR

It's often said that countries' militaries are mired in fighting the last war.

For example, navies build more large ships to combat the memory of the last war's naval battles, which are also the battles projected to come. But the future is not always a repeat of the past and the next threat, perhaps attack by a swarm of small ships, may leave large ships at a decided disadvantage.

So, too, many physician groups are fighting the last war, imagining that the threat to their existence is from, say, the hospital, or from a certain type of other specialists.

But the reality may be very different.

Many of the scenarios that medical groups consider in setting their strategy, if they engage in strategy work at all, and if they consider alternative scenarios at all, are mired in the past: Past battles that were either won or lost, but past all the same.

The pace of change in healthcare is accelerating dramatically. At the same time that the federal government is poised to grab more control through the implementation of Obamacare, so too will some states begin to implement other "reform."

And, at the same time, disruptive providers, hospitals, large employers, new technologies, and entrepreneurial thinkers will change the landscape on which your group's competitiveness will be measured.

It's no longer business as usual. It is business as unusual. And that requires a new way of thinking.

ARE YOU BLINDED BY SUCCESS?

The Rock Solid Group, a fictitious name for what was once a very real group, had a lock on the services that it provided to St. Mark's Community Memorial Hospital, again a disguise for a very real place. And then . . . poof! . . . it all evaporated, leaving the former members of the former group as shocked as if an elephant had disappeared off of an illusionist's stage.

For years, Rock Solid had not only performed well, its owner–physicians earned close to 100% more than what the MGMA would report as 75th percentile compensation.

But what they didn't do when they were riding high, because they were blinded by riding high, was expand their business significantly beyond their relationship with St. Mark's.

They misunderstood the risky place they were in. Sure, the odds that the contract between Rock Solid and St. Mark's Community Memorial would come to a screeching halt were low, but they ignored the fact that low odds times the life changing magnitude of an end to that relationship yields an extremely high risk. Later, of course, that lesson was made all too clear to them.

Medical groups of all shapes, sizes and specialties must take this lesson to heart. Just because things are going well doesn't mean that you don't need to strategize for your future. In fact, when things are going well you are in the best position to strategize for your future.

What potential risks does your group face? Where are you vulnerable? What alternatives and opportunities exist to reduce the risk and vulnerability? Which ones should you pursue? What is the first step in pursuing them?

The processes that I've written about in other posts, including Focus on the Future™, the Strategic Group Process™, and the Scenario Survey Process™ are all tools that you can use, and should use, now.

Just because you don't see a problem on the horizon doesn't mean it doesn't exist. Absence of proof is not proof of absence.

SPARE CHANGE

If you don't like all of this change going on around you in health care, start instituting some change on your own.

Too many physicians think that they don't have any control over the future, but many of the structures they feel trapped in didn't even exist five years ago. Someone created those structures–that is, someone instituted that change.

Prohibitions as to new physician owned Medicare certified hospitals stifling you? Start another type of facility or one that's not aimed at Medicare patients.

Referring physicians pressuring you for a share of your fees (yes, it's illegal)? Your feet aren't cemented, walk.

Complaining, though, won't get you very far.

L'AIR DU TEMPS

It was a breezy day. Dozens of sailboats dotted the sea outside of the safety of the Santa Barbara harbor.

Many were running with the wind, being propelled quickly in the direction chosen by it.

Others were heading, in general but not absolute terms, against it by tacking at angles across it.

L'air du temps, the spirit of the times, in healthcare is not much different from the wind buffeting those sailboats: Communal, "we" not "me," top down not bottom up.

For your medical group to succeed, you need to understand the direction of the societal wind. You might like it. You might hate it. Either way, it's still windy.

Just as the boat captain must deal with the wind, not ignore it, medical group leaders must in any event accept that l'air du temps is real, that it exists.

If you want to go where that wind is pushing you, then go for it and adopt a business strategy in conformity with it. If you find l'air du temps to be polluted, then chart a course across it, not into it.

But in any event, you can't simply allow the wind to buffet against you without navigation, and you can't simply drop sail and pray to be rescued.

Hospital - Central Healthcare

TWO WOLVES AND A LAMB

Benjamin Franklin wrote that democracy is like two wolves and a lamb voting on what to have for lunch; liberty is a well armed lamb contesting the vote.

Hospitals and the government believe that the best way to improve the quality of healthcare is to have more collaboration between physicians and hospitals. But, of course, they're not simply talking about working collaboration, they're talking about financial collaboration. And of course, the hospitals want to be in charge of the purse.

So we have our two wolves and we have physicians, the lambs, deciding on the best way to allocate scarce resources.

Of course there's a bit of a jump in logic here and that's because there's no reason why greater collaboration between physicians and hospitals requires economic collaboration at all.

After all, one of the sentinel events in our business lifetimes has been the change brought about by the invention of the microchip and the ensuing technological advances, all of which have served in our economy in general to break down bureaucratic structures due to the increased ability of individuals and small enterprises to compete and for entrepreneurial activity to coordinate across the membranes of separate business organizations as the results of computerization and related technology.

But to believe the government and hospitals, closer financial integration and closer business integration is what is required in order to deliver quality healthcare.

Of course this is a lie, an attractive lie to be sure. What it's really about is power and control.

Physicians should be all for collaboration in terms of patient care, collaboration with other providers and collaboration with facilities.

But hospitals should play a very small role in that they are, to a large extent, dinosaurs of an earlier era in which close physical proximity and bureaucratic structures were required to compete.

If there are to be collaborative care structures, they should be physician-centric, but this will only happen if the lambs are well armed with knowledge and with political organization and expert assistance.

The two wolves have voted to have lamb for lunch. You are on the menu.

SCHOOL CAFETERIAS. PATIENT CARE.

I'd stand in line to get lunch in the cafeteria. Patrick Henry Junior High.

Enchiladas that were reminiscent of lasagna. Hot dogs that were reminiscent of plastic.

But it was the only food sold on campus. There was no need to make it any better. They had the ultimate competitive advantage for a "restaurant:" A starving crowd.

As hospitals build employed staff models, as they build ACO networks, and as they influence referrals within those "staffs," will the quality of care go up, or will it go down?

At least I could bring my own lunch.

MOVING AWAY FROM BIG . . . EXCEPT IN HEALTHCARE

It's almost 2 pm and I'm hungry and I'm thinking about going to a restaurant for lunch.

But for the last hour or so, instead of thinking about my stomach, I've been thinking about the overall business model of healthcare and how it's changing.

But is it changing for the best?

In almost every area of society, the change is away from big, away from corporate (or at least traditional corporate), toward small.

All courtesy of the microchip.

So, we have Zip car competing with Hertz and Avis and even, for some, with the notion of owning a car at all.

And, we have AirBnB, linking home-sharers with travelers looking for a place to stay, competing with Hilton and Marriott.

And so on.

Yet in healthcare the model is changing in the other direction, toward big, toward hospital-centricity. This is swimming upstream in the river of data and connectivity that enables health information to be shared across independent providers (which is what HIPAA is all about).

The shift toward hospital-centric healthcare can't last. It can't because everything about it runs contrary to society's direction. The only way this won't be true is if it's imposed by force. Oh, I mean by rule of law.

There are some cracks in the system already. Walk in clinics of various stripes. Physician services as cosmetics. Travel medicine. Concierge medicine.

But those ideas are not truly disruptive in the sense of the anxiety that say, Uber is giving to the taxi business.

Why not doctors freely using facilities like performers access concert venues? Why not links among providers like "code sharing" among airlines? Why not individuals sharing healthcare cost risk via crowdsourced risk pools without exchanges or employers? Why not a star system of healthcare providers? Why not boutique hospitals within hotels? Why not offshore health destinations unregulated by national governments?

Well, I'm still hungry but I don't think I'll go to a restaurant. There's a food truck that just pulled to the curb down the block. The restaurants may not like it, but I do.

(So why not mobile hospitals or physicians offices rolling down the street?)

Let me know.

What's your idea?

HOSPITAL CEO GETS A RAISE. YOU? WE'RE NOT SO SURE.

Hey, I've got a great job for you.

A study released earlier this year found little correlation between nonprofit hospitals' CEO pay, which averaged almost $600,000 per year, and performance in respect of charity hospitals' touted values — charity care and mortality rates — or patient care.

What are these people being paid for? Won't someone do it for less?

Why would anyone donate at to a charity if the CEO, who optimally would be either a volunteer or paid at say a high school teacher level, is earning a wasteful salary?

Oh, your job? It's tied to performance in the hospital's ACO. Sorry, the exact number is going to be determined by a committee after the fact. Trust us.

SHOULD HOSPITALS BE PUBLIC UTILITIES?

Would you write a check to a charity that pays its top executive $3 million a year? Does that charity really need your money?

You turn on the faucet and scoop up a cool splash of water onto your face.

How'd the water get to your faucet?

For most, the water got there via a public utility, a regulated business serving all comers. Regulated rates. Run by bureaucrats with bureaucratic salaries. Or, in some places, run as a public department. Again with regulated rates. Run by bureaucrats with bureaucratic salaries.

Recent news reports have revealed that some non-profit hospital CEOs have received up to 40% increases in salary over the prior year, with some CEO's compensation hitting the $3 million mark.

Perhaps all hospitals should be public utilities. Controlled profit. Open not only to all patients at regulated rates, but open to all physicians who qualify for staff privileges. Or, if not public utilities, at least facilities with open medical staffs.

Maybe hospitals as utilities is the wrong approach. Perhaps they should be non-profit cooperatives, with physician members. Or perhaps they should be like state courthouses, open to all licensed physicians in the way that all members of the bar can appear in court. Or what if they continue to operate in the current fashion, but with an absolute prohibition on the corporate practice of medicine — a true wall between healthcare facility and physician?

I don't know how I think about this. I certainly don't believe that the provision of healthcare professional services, as opposed to the factories in which healthcare professional services are sometimes delivered (i.e., hospitals), should be regulated nearly as much as it is now.

So, I'm not lecturing. I'm not even giving my opinion (for once). I'm just thinking out loud.

What do you think?

But something is broken here. I think we should view it as a healthcare crisis. A real one this time.

THE BARS SLAMMED SHUT BEHIND THE DOCTOR

The bars slammed shut behind the doctor.

All he did was order an implantable device for his patient — the device came from a physician owned distributorship, or "POD," in which he held an ownership interest.

On July 26, 2013, the Wall Street Journal ran a page 1 story on a surgeon from Ventura County, California. He's under investigation for improper self referral in connection with his interest in a POD. The facts of this doctor's story are complicated, but the take home point for you is that the viewpoint of the article is indignation that a physician would have an interest in a device.

But where's the indignation over a hospital having an interest in referrals from its facility to physicians employed by it? Where's the indignation over a hospital having an interest in referrals from one employed physician to another?

Yes, I'm aware of Stark and I'm aware of states' companion statues. That's the point.

Why indignation for self interest in one situation but not in its functional equivalent?

There are reasons. And then there is the real reason. So what's the real reason?

PSST, WANNA BUY A WATCH? THE MYTH OF SECURITY IN HOSPITAL EMPLOYMENT

Growing up in the 1960's and early 1970's, it was a common assumption that going to college and getting a job with a large company was the key to financial security. How did that work out for the millions of corporate employees who saw their jobs disappear when their companies failed, when they were laid off in a downsizing (oh, sorry, "right sizing"), or simply replaced by someone who'd work for less?

Today many so-called experts are telling physicians that the key to financial security is in close alignment with – read that as employment by – hospitals.

Do they really think you're that blind?

Sorry, but there is no security, at least nothing absolute, nothing that can be assured you. Large organizations are not more stable than small ones. There are very few, if any economies of scale.

No matter what, you are bearing the risk. Wouldn't you rather hedge your chances by having more control over your destiny?

Being free to practice medicine without the attendant worries of running a business is the recruiting poster for those who want to pay you at the median of last year's salary survey, a continuously decreasing sum.

It's a con, a long con, and you're the mark.

PATIENT COMPLICATIONS PRODUCE HOSPITAL PROFITS

In my April 8, 2013, blog post Amorality Of Institutions – An Additional Argument For Physician Control Of Hospitals, I argued that hospitals, as institutions, are at best amoral. At the same time, they are driven by profit and their executives bear no true downside risk, no risk of going negative in terms of personal liability. Those points, I posit, support the fact that physicians should run hospitals.

And now, more recently, comes a Wall Street Journal article (Treatment Woes Can Bolster Profits, April 17, 2013) revealing that the campaign to battle hospital complications is being slowed by the fact that hospitals profit from patient complications. On top of that, it costs hospitals significant money to reduce complications.

So what we have are institutions that avoid doing the right thing because it will cost them money out of pocket to achieve a result that will cost them far more in prospective profits.

Obviously, what's needed is a counter-weight. I suggested two in my April 8, 2013, post: Make hospital executives and administrators personally liable for their decisions. Shift control of healthcare to physicians, putting hospitals back into the position they occupied when hospitals first came into being.

What do you think?

A TIP ABOUT PHYSICIAN ALIGNMENT

Although, unfortunately, it's too late for physicians to rally against the imposition of Obamacare (but never too late to lend support to those who will repeal it), it's not too late to see that unless physicians plot their own future, the hospitals (and the government and, to the extent they will long exist…that's another topic…health insurers) have a future planned for you.

I've written about the issue of the spiraling down of compensation that's resulting from increased hospital employment of physicians.

On top of that, there's a tipping point reached in a community once a significant number of physicians are "aligned" – the result is that the physicians on the outside of "alignment" don't receive enough referrals and go away, while those on the inside are surely commoditized and can be replaced more easily than ever.

Clinical alignment is a great thing. Complete economic alignment is stupid.

[A shout out to Renee Slater, CPA for the email exchange that led to this posting.]

AMORALITY OF INSTITUTIONS – AN ADDITIONAL ARGUMENT FOR PHYSICIAN CONTROL OF HOSPITALS

In my November 28, 2011, post, All Hospitals Should Be Physician Controlled, I discussed the fact that, as a result of society's current communal tide, the trend toward a "we" society, healthcare is becoming increasingly hospital-centric with looming negative impact.

Keeping that in mind, consider now that people, not institutions, are capable of morality. At best, institutions are amoral. At worst, they are immoral.

This doesn't necessarily mean that hospital executives are amoral or immoral in the conduct of their personal lives, or whether they don't have good intentions in their work lives. What it does mean is that institutions—corporations and other entities, whether their tax status is for profit or nonprofit—must make a profit or otherwise meet financial targets in order to continue to survive. The executives get significant salaries and great bonuses if they deliver profit and, at worst, lose bonuses or (sometimes) their jobs if they fail.

But in no case does a hospital executive go truly at risk…at no point does he or she have to dip into his or her personal funds, or declare bankruptcy, if their decisions lead to loss. This is true in terms of the overall push to make a profit and in terms of the impact of withholding care, of cutting corners, of doing just enough but no more.

Individuals, physicians in this discussion, are capable of morality and my experience is that most are highly moral. Sure, there are some bad apples, there are in any subset of society. But no matter where Dr. X lies on moral scale, he or she is ultimately liable for his or her decisions, for his or her actions.

Who would you rather empower to make decisions affecting your personal health: An individual truly at risk, someone with "skin in the game," or an institution that one way or another restricts its employees' actions, led by executives whose chances of suffering from bad decisions are seldom negative at all, and whose most likely ultimate risk is capped at the loss of a bonus?

There are several solutions. One is make hospital executives and administrators personally liable for their decisions. Another is to shift control of healthcare to physicians, putting hospitals back into the position they occupied when hospitals first came into being.

Care to weigh in on this?

TOP DOWN HEALTHCARE IS KILLING YOUR BUSINESS AND (LITERALLY) KILLING YOU AND ME

For hundreds of years, innovation has driven improvement in medicine. Innovation in patient care. Innovation in business models. Innovation in treatment.

Dramatic innovation requires a chaotic marketplace—a marketplace for business as well as a marketplace for ideas.

Conformity is innovation's enemy.

Now take a look at the following visual:

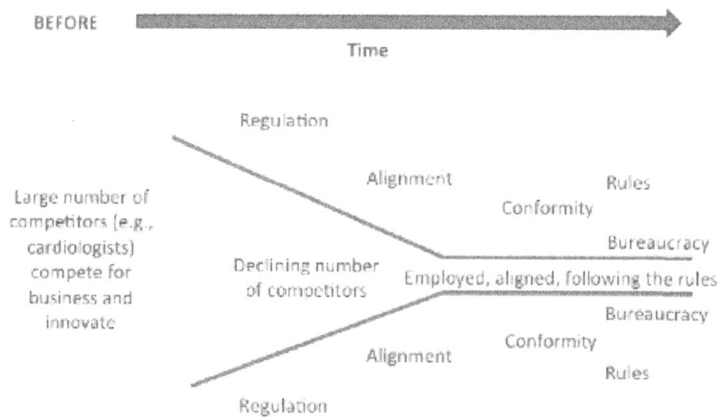

On the left side, you see the situation before ObamaCare. There are multiple competitors in the market—here, in our example, cardiologists. In order to succeed, they had to deliver a better experience to their referral sources, they had to deliver a better experience to their patients, and they had to develop high levels of medical expertise. This required innovation across the board, not simply doing the minimum required to keep their doors open.

As we move toward the right on the visual, with increasing regulation and, importantly with the increasing pressure to align with hospitals, joining ACOs and even becoming employees of hospitals and their affiliates, there are fewer competitors. Those fewer competitors have less reason, and less freedom, to innovate. In order to keep their jobs they must conform. They are now factory workers in someone else's healthcare factory. The fact that the funnel-like image can be rotated 90 degrees clockwise and appear similar to a meat grinder is not unintentional.

So what happens to innovation? What happens to excellence?

Sorry, but I don't believe for a moment that medicine will attract the same level of interest among high achievers 20 years from now unless there is a radical change. It might be possible to make more as a plumber. There certainly will be more freedom.

None of this is good for your business. None of this is good for your health, or mine. But the bureaucrats will be able to measure things. They'll know whether you gave an antibiotic at the "right" time. They'll know how many hours you worked. They'll measure whether you gave test "A" before test "B."

The bureaucrats will have exabytes of data on measurable stuff. But the important things, the really important things, will be ignored because they can't be measured – take, for example, innovation that never occurs.

Over the next several months I'll post entries on this topic including strategies to opt out of the serfdom that those bureaucrats who (they think) are smarter than you have in store for your future.

PHYSICIAN SUBSIDIARY ENTITY – ALIGNED OR A'LYING?

The physician subsidiary entity is a physician alignment model sold as a kinder, gentler, freer alternative to direct hospital employment.

But is it kinder, gentler or freer?

Although there are various alternatives to setting up the subsidiary model, generally the assets of a medical group are sold to the hospital. Then either the physicians formerly engaged by the medical group remain as employees of the group, which is now owned by a physician "friendly" to the hospital, or they become employees of a new professional corporation owned by the hospital-friendly physician.

The notion is that although the hospital essentially owns the group, the group's physicians, subject to rights retained by the hospital, control the medical group's board of directors. Purportedly, this provides the physicians with greater autonomy including determining how compensation is allocated among them.

But, as all compensation to the group is either flowing directly from the hospital or is metered by it, query whether that control is real or illusory.

The physicians do have more control over how the allowed sum is allocated among them (or, at least the board or the officers of the subsidiary hold that control) but it's a fallacy that the subsidiary has any real existence beyond that. The upside has been completely capped.

Of course, if the only two alternatives to be considered are hospital employment with no more group to have a role in determining compensation or an illusory group that permits control physicians to still determine who in the "group" gets what, then there is perhaps more "freedom" in the latter model.

It's the same degree of freedom that exists within the giraffe enclosure at the Santa Barbara Zoo: the giraffes can run anywhere they want, except where they can't.

EMPLOYMENT INSECURITY

Have they got a deal for you.

As a physician, you're concerned about increasing competition, declining reimbursement, and, of course, the looming impact of Obamacare.

So, you've been thinking, as have many, many of your colleagues, that it's time to give up independent practice, whether truly solo practice or as a member of a group. There's so much more security in hospital employment and a regular paycheck. Or so you and they think.

But what security is there in an agreement with a one or two year term? Or even a 7 year term…with a 60 or 90 day termination without cause provision? There is none.

Across the country, employees in many industries are just days away from a layoff or termination. Or, because they have no control over the decision, they fear that they are, which is just as bad.

Hospital employment? Sure, it's security . . . in some alternative universe.

Comment or contact me if you'd like to discuss this post.

DOES YOUR GROUP OWN ITS FUTURE OR ARE YOU MERELY RENTING IT?

Henry grew his restaurant from a shack selling hot dogs into a wildly successful business generating an incredible profit. It took years of labor, great service, and development of superb relationships with customers.

Then it ended.

You see, the restaurant was Henry's sole business. And, it was located smack dab in the middle of a county fairground.

The fact that the county leased the facility out multiple times each week for large events which drew tens or even hundreds of thousands of people, most of whom where hungry and who had no option of eating somewhere else on the grounds, was no longer of any consequence when the county refused to renew Henry's contract and, in essence, gave his business to a new "vendor."

In reality, Henry never really owned his business. He was simply its caretaker. He just realized it a bit too late. In essence, this is the same situation many hospital-based groups have created for themselves. Their entire business is, in essence, located on "leased space," that is, at a single hospital. And, that lease is probably abysmally short, it might even be subject to termination at any time on 90 days notice.

And soon, due to the wave of financial alignment with hospitals, office-based specialists will increasingly be in the same boat.

More and more hospitals are more and more upfront about the vendor status they have placed you in. Even if you resisted expansion of your business for years out of some misplaced notion that you would be poaching on your colleagues down the road, pay attention to the lesson of Henry and his restaurant: It was a concession stand — just as is, in many hospital administrators' minds, your practice.

Whose mind will be easier to change, the administrator's about your vendor status or your own about the need to strategize, and then act, to preserve your future?

GRAND THEFT AUTO

When I was 14, my friend Steve and I were stopped by the police for breaking into a car.

We didn't actually break into a car. We just walked past it in the parking lot on our way into a store. The cop just decided to hassle us. His idea of fun, maybe. At least he became a cop and not a criminal.

The other day, I heard a potential client tell me that his future was being stopped.

The hospital administrator had told him that if he doesn't stop pushing to expand the scope of his group's exclusive contract, the group would be "fired."

No one's future is really dependent upon the approval of someone else. This guy I'm talking about, this doctor, may have painted himself and his group into a corner: the hospital might be the only facility at which they work. But that was his doing, not someone else's.

And, even if they are painted into a corner, they can always bust out through the wall. Take their show on the road, so to speak. But no one ever really thinks of that. If you structure your group correctly, it's entirely possible. Of course, it would be better to be working at multiple facilities so that if one is no longer desirable to you, you can tell them to take a hike.

This guy's group really has no future at that place. The reality is that the hospital administrator really has no place to go. He's just got a job and when he's fired he'll have a harder time finding a new position than you anyway. Or, maybe he won't be fired. Maybe he'll get some award for cutting costs. Maybe. But who wants to work with a jerk like him, anyway?

Back when I was 14, I thought that that cop was a criminal. A child abuser. Maybe he was.

Group Culture

THE MISMATCH OF STORY AND CULTURE WITHIN MEDICAL GROUPS

I had a friend, let's call him "Bob," who'd readily make promises and just as readily break them.

All medical groups have a culture, whether or not it's been purposefully created. It exists.

All medical groups have a story, too. A story its leaders or members or both tell about the group.

So, while culture exists, story itself is a representation or image of culture.

Some say that story is how culture is transmitted. But what I'd like you to focus on is the impact of the match or mismatch between story and culture within a medical group and how it affects the group both internally and externally.

The Community Group prides itself on delivering high quality care and on meeting the needs of its patients and referring physicians. That's the story they tell themselves.

If that story matches with the actual culture, that is, the group actually delivers high quality care that meets its customers' needs, then value is being created for the customers and it's likely that the group is highly performing internally.

On the other hand, if the story remains the same but the group's physicians are rude and if reports promised to referring physicians are generally late, then there's trouble in store for the group — they are just fooling themselves and no one else.

The same mismatch can happen internally as well. For example, when a group's leaders believe (belief being the story) that they have created a culture of mentoring younger group members but the reality is that there is no guidance and that management by yelling around is the rule. That misalignment of story and culture creates a cancer within the group.

My friend Bob thought that he was a man of his word. But that was just a story.

I WANT TO BECOME A PARTNER

"I want to become a partner."

Lawyers hear this all the time from newer members of their firm. Doctors, too, hear it from junior members of their medical group.

Partnership is, it appears, the Holy Grail that, once grasped, results in eternal professional success.

But what does partnership really mean? People focus on the upside, or, actually, the imagined upside. They rarely stop to wonder what that upside might actually be. And they rarely, if ever, focus on the downside: the liability and the responsibility that comes with ownership.

I once had a partner who commented that it would be cheaper to make Bob, not his real name, a partner because we could then pay him less.

That comment triggers at least two thoughts: First, there may be tremendous problems in a professional practice if it cannot distribute a greater reward to its owners than to its employees. And second, "partnership" in some instances might be some type of scam.

Be careful about what you wish for. Those holding the keys to your "success" might be all too willing to hand them over to you.

DOES YOUR EMPLOYMENT CONTRACT HAVE TEETH?

Your practice has worked hard to expand to a second location or a third or a fourth. These can be other ASCs at which your group provides anesthesia, satellite offices for your cardiology group, or additional G.I. centers for your gastroenterology practice — the story runs across all medical specialties.

But what happens when one of the members of your group who is assigned to work at different sites, acts out on his or her bias against working at a particular location, perhaps by showing up late, or by making untoward comments to the staff, or by engaging in some other type of disruptive behavior?

The answer, of course, is that slowly but surely it begins to destroy your business opportunities. An anesthesiologist showing up late at a surgery center can be the beginning of the end of your group's entire relationship with that facility. The cardiologist who doesn't like working at your satellite office in the suburbs can easily telegraph this to referring physicians, drying up streams of business.

Certainly, there are personnel, management, and contractual issues involved. But on the purely contractual side, your practice's employment agreement or subcontract agreement with physicians must either delineate level of service expectations or make reference to policies and procedures that must be complied with. And your group must have "teeth" to enforce compliance as well as the will to do so.

Practices fall apart from the inside more often than most realize.

Take the time to analyze the contractual protections your group has developed, or hasn't developed, now, before you need to start looking at what you can enforce.

DOES YOUR GROUP'S COMPENSATION PLAN SUFFER FROM THIS DEFECT?

There's a management saying that what's measured improves. As a result, managers love to measure things. But measuring does not always indicate value.

Take for example a family of three with total income of $200,000 a year. The parents have another child. Should grandma call the parents to commiserate because the family's per capita income just dropped from $66,666 to $50,000?

So clearly, you've got to be measuring the right thing.

The family comedy described above has a medical group analogy. Groups must distinguish between measuring things which are efficient and measuring things which create a much improved or larger experience for the recipient.

What if you were running a restaurant instead of a medical group. Let's say you decide to measure and reward on the basis of the time a waiter or waitress takes to picks up food in the kitchen and deliver it to the table. Soon, waiters would be jogging through the joint, tossing plates onto the tables. Slopping the food onto the table with a smirk would still be 99th percentile performance, but the total customer experience would be at rock bottom.

So clearly, some things that measurement says are now "improved" aren't anything of the sort.

Now back to running a medical group. Take a look at your group's compensation plan. If you simply measure units produced by your group members–that is, you pay by units only–then you are encouraging fast delivery, not courteous service: tossing the plates, so to speak. On the other hand, if you've adopted a fixed compensation system, $X per month as salary, you've taken away the incentive to work harder, and you've ignored the notion of an incentive for better performance. Of course, that still begs the question, what is better performance?

Correctly formulated, a group compensation plan is not just about encouraging efficiency, it's about encouraging effective performance in a broad sense. Some of that performance is capable of meaningful objective measurement, but a significant portion is not — but that portion can't be ignored, it still has to be considered and group members must be cognizant of its impact on their overall compensation.

WHO IS REALLY IN CHARGE OF YOUR MEDICAL GROUP?

Some leaders of hospital-based groups, and I use the term "leader" broadly, believe that their groups are a function of the hospital. If the hospital no longer wants to contract with them, then that would be it, they'd simply pulled the plug on the group.

But what kind of group is that? What kind of leader is that? What kind of business is that?

Sure, Peter Drucker is quoted as stating the purpose of business is to create and keep a customer, but I he wasn't speaking in the singular, i.e., a single customer.

If a group allows itself to get into that position, then it has truly lost control of its business function. In fact, it's allowed itself to become simply a risk taker – in essence managing the risk of providing its type of specialty services for the hospital. The group takes the risk of recruitment, of coverage, of collections, of having necessary cash flow to pay its providers, etc. But the hospital really runs the business as it controls the group's future.

What kind of future is that?

THE ADVANTAGE IS TO . . .

Speed and size are often an advantage, but in some situations, and in some markets, they're not. For medical groups, the current healthcare market is one of them.

For example, pointing to the work of John Boyd, speed alone in terms of fighter jets isn't the key; it's speed, plus maneuverability, plus the ability to quickly increase and quickly decrease speed. Similarly, we're all familiar with the concept of the inability of a large ship to change direction quickly.

For entrepreneurial medical groups, relatively smaller size can be a tremendous advantage in an uncertain and unclear market. That's the market we're in now.. But that's only the case if the group's leadership has in place the governance structure to enable it to make and implement decisions quickly. And of course, that's only the case if those in leadership roles have the time, ability and inclination to actually exercise their power.

How maneuverable is your group? Titanic heading for an iceberg or highly maneuverable speedboat?

DISRUPTIVE PHYSICIAN – YOU KNOW WHO! (HE/SHE WORKS FOR YOU)

I hated taking out the trash.

When I was a kid, my parents' garbage cans were in a little yard next to the garage. Mondays were "trash day" and that meant that on Sunday night, when I was already dreading going back to school the next morning, I also had to dread taking out the trash. I mean it really stunk. Like old fish. And old chicken. And dog stuff, too.

But I had to take it out.

When you think of a medical group failing, you often think that a competitor crushed them. That's sometimes what happened. But often the rot started from within — a disruptive or megalomaniacal or bad-mouthing group member.

Benjamin Franklin is said to have quipped that house guests and fish smell after three days. Crappy group members stink a lot faster than that.

Sure, it's all PC to "counsel" these guys. To tell them how much you love them if only they will toe the line and be good boys or girls and get along with everyone while singing Kumbaya.

Go ahead, try it once. But after that, realize that these people just can't help themselves. In your group they are a rot that will spread. In some other setting they may be perfectly happy, highly productive good citizens. Do them a favor and get them started on their journey to find their perfect spot: it is somewhere else. Fire them.

The corollary is that you must make certain that your group's contracts, your employment agreement, partnership agreement or other applicable agreements, create the ability to save your group from this rot.

It's Sunday night for your group. Time to take out the trash.

YOU DESERVE IT

There's a simple meme, an idea that spreads, in today's society, one that advertisers are keen to exploit: The "deserve it" meme.

"It's the [advertiser: fill this in] that you deserve!"

Unfortunately, this meme impacts medical group thinking as well. As in "we deserve the exclusive contract," or "I deserve her referrals."

Just as Mr. Jones is fooling himself when he believes he actually deserves that Obama phone, Dr. Jones is fooling herself when she believes that her group's exclusive contract will simply be renewed and renewed and renewed because it is "deserved." Or because it's "fair." Or because that's the way that it's always been.

One key to actually getting what you want is providing value to the one you want it from. Another is negotiating agreements with longer terms and not-so-easy-to-trigger termination provisions.

But this all starts with adopting a mindset that runs counter to the trending meme: "I don't deserve it (in the entitlement sense), so how am I going to get it and how am I going to keep it?"

That's a strategic mindset.

So, as they say on TV, start now and get the future you deserve

Competing Against Yourself

THE PRESIDENT AND THE "NO-STORM"

A few minutes ago, CNN told me that the president didn't actually sell out to the Iranians and that a killer storm is hitting Dallas.

The pilot of the plane I'm now on, headed to Dallas, says we'll have a smooth flight: the storm never materialized.

Who's telling your medical group a story? Do you believe it?

What story might you be telling, if even (no, especially) to yourself?

IT'S NOT WHAT YOU SAID, IT'S HOW YOU SAID IT

"Mark, it's not what you said, it's how you said it."

When I was a kid, my father said that to me all the time.

It's all about the unspoken message.

Last week, I spoke at the AICPA's national healthcare conference. It was at The Roosevelt Hotel in New Orleans, a Hilton under the Waldorf Astoria brand. Here's how they greet you:

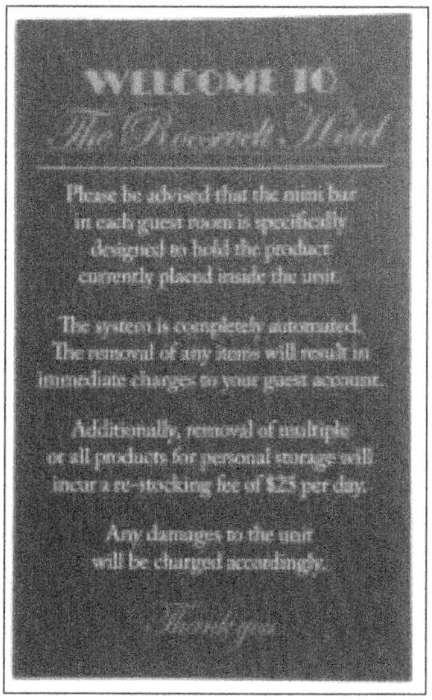

Welcome…please be advised…we're too lazy to actually see if you actually took that candy bar, so if you move it out of the mini bar to check to see if it's got peanuts in it, we'll charge you immediately…thank you.

How would you feel if you were invited to a dinner party and when the host greets you at the door he hands you the house rules?

What's really being communicated? That the Hilton folks are lazy idiots who have no concept of customer service?

What's really being said in your physicians' interactions with patients, with referring physicians, and with hospital administrators?

That you really don't care if your patients are reading a two year old magazine while they sit on their asses for 45 minutes in your waiting room. That Mrs. Smith is a number not a valued customer, so the first communication she receives from your group is a bill?

Are your group's physicians smiling in the hospital hallway while really communicating indifference, or worse, contempt?

Sooner or later, the real message gets through. It gets through right to your group's financial bottom line.

THE CAT'S AWAY. THE MICE DID PLAY. MEDICAL GROUP R.I.P.

It was the late 1970's.

The owner of the physician network, one of the earliest managed care entities on the West Coast, was based outside of the country. His business was managed by U.S. based employees.

So, while the cat was away, the mice did play.

Like one of those episodes of a restaurant spy camera show, you know, where they catch the employees of the Italian restaurant running a Mexican food joint from the place on the owner's day off, the U.S. based managers plotted their own venture. Then they pulled it off.

Similar coups and business cloning often decimate medical groups, both office based and hospital based practices.

The lessons:

1. Hire the right employees.
2. If you trust, you must still verify.
3. You can't be a completely absentee "owner." Absent can mean being across the ocean, across the country, or even, in my experience, two floors up the elevator shaft.

4. If enforceable in the jurisdiction, include covenants not to compete in your employment agreements, subcontracts, and ownership documents, e.g., the partnership agreement.
5. In all jurisdictions, include other protective provisions in your deals.

You've built your practice. If you do what I recommend, you've expanded its operations.

Now protect it.

STOP TRADE SECRETS FROM WALKING OUT THE DOOR

Your medical group's most important assets, its physicians and other providers, walk out the door each night.

What are they carrying with them?

Take the Viceroy group (not its real name), for example. Yes, literally take it. At least that's what several of its owners did when they jumped ship to a competitor which then displaced Viceroy as the holder of its exclusive contract.

It's great to develop team spirit and camaraderie to hold a group together. But it's not enough to rely on it to protect your group's sensitive data and strategies.

Trade secret provisions must be incorporated into your group's services agreements and its partnership/shareholders agreements. But for those provisions to be effective, trade secrets must actually be guarded and closely held.

In states where they are enforceable, use covenants not to compete. In jurisdictions where those covenants are not enforceable (and even where they are), other restrictions, some common and others proprietary, can be used to dissuade a group physician from leaving to compete.

What's your group's practice worth? Make the investment to protect it.

TAKEN THE WRONG JOB?

I knew that I had taken the wrong job after my first day at the firm.

More than thirty years have passed, so now I can laugh about it. But back then, I thought I was screwed.

The majority of the partners were probably geniuses, but they had little, if any human characteristics.

Perhaps they were cyborgs. I'm really not sure.

Have you made this same mistake? Either by taking a job with idiot savants or, even worse yet, by building a medical group comprised of them?

The rationalization is that are "great doctors." Or that they have CVs as thick as the phone book. But they destroy your group's relationships with "customers" of all stripes: referral sources, patients, hospitals, coworkers.

It's like a great mechanic who smokes in your car. I had one once and never went back.

My old bosses made another mistake. They pissed off clients and didn't do anything to protect their business.

Watch out who you work for. If they're jerks, plan on how to obtain the benefit they are unknowingly passing along to you.

If you're a group leader, watch out for who you hire. Take precautions that they don't destroy your practice's relationships. Have the contractual ability to discipline and terminate.

Me, I stayed long enough not to damage my resume and then began looking for a new job. The cyborgs found out and fired me before I could give notice. I took a huge book of business with me to my new firm. To this day, I am grateful to them.

Changing Market

HOW SOON WILL HIJACKED FAIRNESS BE COMING TO HEALTHCARE?

In places where fairness is judged by outcome, not opportunity, it soon takes on a surreal twist. Take France, for example. Or maybe Sacramento.

The Wall Street Journal reported earlier this year that Sephora, the cosmetic chain, has been told by the French courts that it can no longer keep its flagship Paris store, on the Champs-Elysees, open past 9:00 p.m. Why? It wouldn't be fair to the workers.

The 58 store employees working the late shift are protesting – against the closure order - they like working the late shift.

And Sephora, which has almost as many visitors per year at their Champs-Elysees store as does the Eiffel Tower, around 3 million, does 20% of its business after 9:00 p.m. It may have to lay off 45 employees if it is forced to close early.

You see, the union and the government do not like the idea of workers, any workers, being made to work late. It's not good for "the social fabric of the family." Even if the workers working late like it. Even if the employer can only employ them because of nighttime sales.

In the top down world, there is a disincentive to get ahead. Caps and controls and, as Sephora has seen, courts.

There's tremendous pressure in that world pushing down those that want to get ahead, those that don't simply want to be mediocre, those that bridle at the notion of just being good enough to collect a paycheck but no more.

As healthcare becomes more consolidated, especially in terms of the growing hospital-centric "alignment" of physicians, will physician unions, those that already exist or new ones, begin to demand that physicians be treated "fairly?" Eight, or perhaps six, hour workdays. No weekends, of course. No more physician abuse. Will doctors in the United States, as they have done in Canada, picket in front of hospitals wearing their white lab coats?

What's the real cost to society? What's the real cost to your self esteem?

MIXED MESSAGE: RESTRICTING SCOPE OF PRACTICE AT MEDI-SPAS, INCREASING IT ELSEWHERE

I read an article in the Wall Street Journal reporting that more states are regulating Medi-Spa ownership and placing scope of practice restrictions on the procedures performed at those facilities.

It seems as if they've discovered that nurses and other paraprofessionals, and in some cases, even beauticians, are performing what many, most, or, perhaps, nearly all, physicians would say are medical procedures.

So, states are rushing to regulate: In some locations, physicians must own or control the spa, and in other cases, states are making sure that physicians actually supervise these procedures.

Yet, in the loony world in which these states regulate, many are also rushing to expand the scope of practice of paraprofessionals in the traditional healthcare setting, e.g., office practice and at the hospital, due to the existing, and soon to be worse, physician shortage resulting from Obamacare.

So, on the one hand, your tattoo may have to be removed by a physician, but your appendectomy might be performed by a nurse practitioner. Go figure.

On the one hand, there's good news here: Physicians pulling out of traditional practice will soon be able to open a Medi-Spa with less competition from those pesky beauticians and allied health professionals.

I feel better, don't you?

NEW OIG ADVISORY OPINION 13-15 SHEDS FURTHER LIGHT ON COMPANY MODEL TYPE ARRANGEMENTS

[Disclosure: I am the attorney for the anesthesia group which was the Requestor of Advisory Opinion 13-15 and represented it in connection with its Request.]

On November 12, 2013, the Office of Inspector General ("OIG") of the Department of Health and Human Services publicly released the redacted version of its Advisory Opinion 13-15. Although the fact pattern is not completely on point with the standard "company model" deal, and is far more complex, it sheds light on the limits of those arrangements.

In particular, the proposed arrangement involved placing the referring physician/medical group in the position of capturing the difference between the amount collected and a per diem rate to be paid to the anesthesia provider.

The OIG declined to approve the arrangement.

The Opinion also questions the legality of a carve out provision in an anesthesia exclusive contract in favor of the referring medical group.

The Facts

The Requestor is an anesthesia group.

From 1993 until early 2011, the anesthesia group contracted with a hospital ("Hospital") to provide all anesthesia services, other than chronic pain management procedures, on an exclusive basis. The scope of the exclusive contract therefore included anesthesia services for ECT procedures performed at the Hospital.

In late 2010, a medical group ("Psychiatry Group") with a medical practice centering on performing electroconvulsive therapy ("ECT") procedures relocated to the Hospital. One of the owners of Psychiatry Group is Dr. X, who is board certified in both psychiatry and anesthesiology but who no longer accepts new psychiatry patients.

Shortly after the Psychiatry Group relocated to the Hospital, the anesthesia group began negotiating the 2011 renewal of its exclusive anesthesia service contract (the "2011 Contract") with the Hospital. In the course of negotiating the 2011 Contract, the Hospital negotiated for Dr. X's right to provide anesthesia services to ECT patients independent of any relationship with Requestor. The anesthesia group attempted to negotiate out of that carve out, but the Hospital refused: The final 2011 Contract included a provision permitting Dr. X to provide anesthesia services to ECT patients in the Hospital's ECT program and requiring the anesthesia group to provide up to six weeks of coverage for Dr. X for ECT procedures that otherwise would have been performed by Dr. X in his role as an anesthesiologist. That 2011 Contract had a one-year term.

Subsequently, in the course of negotiating the 2012 renewal of the anesthesia services contract (the "2012 Contract"), the Hospital negotiated for further amendments to the 2011 Contract's carve-out provision. Ultimately, the 2012 Contract allowed Dr. X to provide anesthesia services to ECT patients in the Hospital's ECT program and required the anesthesia group to provide coverage for Dr. X with prior notice as agreed to between the anesthesia group and Dr. X.

The 2012 Contract also included the following provision (the "Additional Anesthesiologist Provision"):

"In the event [the Psychiatry Group] or the Hospital determines that an additional anesthesiologist is needed to provide ECT, [anesthesia group] shall negotiate in good faith with [the Psychiatry Group] to contract with [anesthesia group] to provide those services. If, after good faith negotiations, [anesthesia group] and [the Psychiatry Group] are not successful in negotiating the terms of an agreement for [anesthesia group] to provide anesthesia services to [the Psychiatry Group], then, so long as the last offer from [the Psychiatry Group] was at a fair market value rate, as reasonably determined by the Hospital, [the Psychiatry Group] or [Dr. X] may contract with an additional anesthesiologist to provide anesthesia services for ECT, and the provision of anesthesia services by that additional anesthesiologist shall not constitute a violation of [anesthesia group's right to provide anesthesia services on an exclusive basis]."

Subsequently, the Psychiatry Group informed the anesthesia group that it had determined that an additional part-time physician was needed to provide ECT anesthesia services and asked the anesthesia group to enter into the arrangement examined by the OIG in the Opinion (the "Proposed Arrangement").

Under the Proposed Arrangement, the anesthesia group and the Psychiatry Group would enter into a contract pursuant to which the anesthesia group would fulfill the Psychiatry Group's need for an additional part-time physician to provide ECT anesthesia services: (i) every Monday, (ii) as necessary to provide vacation coverage for Dr. X, and (iii) as necessary when emergent coverage is required. The Psychiatry Group estimated that such coverage would require between 6 and 12 hours of the anesthesiologists' time during each day of service. The anesthesia group would reassign its right to bill for the services rendered by its anesthesiologists to the Psychiatry Group on coverage days. The Psychiatry Group would bill and collect for those services and, in turn, would pay the anesthesia group a fixed, per diem rate of $Y for the anesthesiologists' services, which the anesthesia group maintains is below fair market value and below what it would receive if it billed for the services directly. The Psychiatry Group would retain the difference between the amount collected and the per diem rate.

OIG's Analysis

The OIG has stated on numerous occasions its view that the opportunity to generate a fee could constitute illegal remuneration under the anti-kickback statute, even if no payment is made for a referral. Under the Proposed Arrangement, the anesthesia group would provide the Psychiatry Group the opportunity to generate a fee equal to the difference between the amounts the Psychiatry Group would bill and collect.

The Proposed Arrangement would not qualify for protection under the safe harbor for personal services and management contracts for a number of reasons, including that the aggregate compensation to be paid over the term of the agreement would be neither set in advance nor consistent with fair market value.

In any event, that safe harbor protects only those payments made by a principal (here, the Psychiatry Group) to an agent (here, the anesthesia group); no safe harbor would protect the remuneration the anesthesia group would provide to the Psychiatry Group by way of the discount between the per diem rate and the amount that would actually be collected.

Because failure to comply with a safe harbor does not mean that an arrangement is per se illegal, the OIG then went into an analysis to determine whether, given all of the relevant facts, the Proposed Arrangement would pose no more than a minimal risk under the anti-kickback statute.

The OIG flatly stated that the Proposed Arrangement appears to be designed to permit the Psychiatry Group to do indirectly what it cannot do directly; that is, to receive compensation, in the form of a portion of the anesthesia group's revenues, in return for the Psychiatry Group's referrals of ECT patients to the anesthesia group for anesthesia services.

The Additional Anesthesiologist Provision gave the Psychiatry Group the ability to solicit this remuneration for its ECT patient referrals by allowing the Psychiatry Group to contract with an anesthesiologist other than the anesthesia group if the anesthesia group and the Psychiatry Group were not successful in negotiating the terms of an agreement for the anesthesia group to provide ECT anesthesia services. The Proposed Arrangement therefore presents the significant risk that the remuneration the anesthesia group would provide to the Psychiatry Group—i.e., the opportunity to generate a fee equal to the difference between the amounts the Psychiatry Group would bill and collect for the anesthesia group's services, and the per diem amounts the Psychiatry Group would pay to the anesthesia group —would be in return for the Psychiatry Group's anesthesia referrals.

The OIG concluded that the Proposed Arrangement could potentially generate prohibited remuneration under the anti-kickback statute and that the OIG could potentially impose administrative sanctions in connection with the Proposed Arrangement.

On another important point, although not officially within the scope of the opinion, the OIG noted the problematic nature of the carve out by stating that they cannot exclude the possibility that: (i) the Hospital agreed to negotiate for the Additional Anesthesiologist Provision in exchange for, or to reward, the Psychiatry Group's continued referral of patients to the Hospital for ECT procedures; (ii) the Hospital leveraged its control over its large base of anesthesia referrals to induce the anesthesia group to agree to the Additional Anesthesiologist Provision; and (iii) the anesthesia group agreed to the Additional Anesthesiologist Provision in exchange for access to the Hospital's stream of anesthesia referrals.

Bottom Line Analysis

Advisory Opinion 13-15 is important for several reasons.

First, it once again demonstrates a fact lost to many when discussing "company model" and similar potential anti-kickback law violations: they generally do not fit into an available safe harbor — the personal services and the employment safe harbors. Not only is this because payment to the referral-receiving physician is not set in advance and will vary with the value or volume of referrals, but even more fundamentally because those safe harbors only apply to payments **from** the principal to the agent, not to payments **from** the agent **to** the principal. In 13-15, the discount that permits the referral source to profit from the arrangement is a payment to the principal.

Second, although failure to fit within a safe harbor is not ipso facto fatal, the OIG has again illustrated, as it did, for example, in Advisory Opinion 11-03 and in Advisory Opinion 12-06, that being put in a position to profit from one's referrals raises significant concerns of prohibited remuneration — that is, of violation of the federal anti-kickback statute.

Third, even though it is addressed only in a footnote, the OIG discusses the potential kickback nature underpinning a hospital's carve out from an exclusive contract. Although this issue is distinct from that of company model type ventures and even from the normal circumstance in which anti-kickback analysis often arises, in my experience there are many problematic arrangements centering around hospitals benefiting financially, directly or indirectly, as a result of exclusive contract arrangements and from special carve outs from those arrangements.

Anyone considering entering into an arrangement that potentially violates the federal anti-kickback law should obtain counsel well-versed in the intricacies of the subject.

BURGERS MUST BE BURGERS, BUT DOCTORS MIGHT JUST NOT BE PHYSICIANS

"When I use a word," Humpty Dumpty said, in rather a scornful tone, "it means just what I choose it to mean — neither more nor less." – From Through The Looking Glass by Lewis Carroll.

***

Let's say you're running a restaurant and because you'll only pay your meat supplier $100 a week for hamburger, all he delivers is 50 lbs. of the stuff. But you need 100 lbs. to meet the demand of your customers. What do you do? Do you go out and buy 50 lbs. of textured soy protein and pass it off has hamburger? You'd be tossed in jail.

But recently, hardly anyone even yawned when the State of California announced that it was considering expanding the scope of paraprofessional practice because there weren't enough physicians to go around. Perhaps, the bureaucrats floated, nurse practitioners could practice independently? Perhaps other healthcare licensees could also practice well beyond the scope currently permitted? And with a Ph.D. as the terminal degree in many of these fields, they'll be doctors.

Not enough hamburger? Mix in soy. Not enough physicians? Let others perform many of the same services – we'll just call them all providers, or better yet, doctors.

Look, I'm not belittling the role of non-physicians in healthcare professions, I'm just saying that they're not physicians.

Was restricting to physicians certain areas of practice simply a scam? Were the years of training given to physicians simply a scam? Was patient health what was really being protected?

Was the State of California lying to its citizens before, or is it lying to them now?

One thing hasn't change though: mix your hamburger with soy protein and you're off to jail. After all, a burger must still be a burger.

VENEZUELA, RICE FARMERS AND DOCTORS IN DALLAS

Models. No, not the skinny kind in a magazine. But conceptual frameworks. Like global warming "models" or even Obamacare.

According to a recent Wall Street Journal article, U.S. rice farmers are raking it in on exports to Venezuela. Chavez's legacy of socialism, in which large farms were nationalized, broken up and "redistributed," together with food price controls resulted in the destruction of its farming industry. Similar top down management ruined the beef, coffee, steel and sugar industries.

Humans are complex. Our interactions are complex. Outside of basic urges, like the drive to survive, we can't, especially on a large scale, be modeled by policy wonks and other useless idiots.

Those who are surprised that employers are increasingly turning to part time workers and temps to escape Obamacare are clueless.

Those who think that ACOs and hospital-centric healthcare have a long term survival rate are equally blind.

The key for doctors in Dallas and Des Moines and Detroit, and across the country, is to develop strategy that increases your chances of professional and economic survival in both the likely short lived hospital-centric world and in the physician-patient centric one to follow.

Those in favor of Obamacare claim they did it to help the uninsured. Chavez and the Chavistas claimed that they took the steps they did to help the disenfranchised. But the disenfranchised have become even more so and everyone is suffering.

FOR WHOM ARE HOSPITALS BUILT?

For whom are hospitals built?

For the health of patients or for the financial health and convenience of its operators and staff?

For anyone who's been a patient at both a large, acute care hospital and at a customer-centric facility, for example, at a surgery center, there is often, very often, no comparison in the overall experience.

I'm not saying that some, as in the case of very ill patients or those requiring broad resources to be diagnosed, don't belong in what are today large, general acute care hospitals. However, advances in technology make it possible to either scale-down the size of facilities or to bring services to the patient.

The future does not bode well for large hospitals. Instead, just as those operators need government restrictions on the establishment of smaller, customer service oriented physician owned hospitals, they will soon be battling competitors who will transform delivery to a patient centered scale.

Soon, the patient centered "medical home" might just be the patient's home.

How is your practice going to cope with that? Start strategizing now.

LIFE IS EASY WHEN YOU'VE GIVEN SOMEONE ELSE THE POWER TO DETERMINE YOUR FUTURE

Have you ever been forced into something? Something you hated? Something you really did not want to do? Something that you'd almost give everything up not to have to do?

Market consolidation – that's what's impacting medical groups of all stripes and sizes. Hospital wants to employ you. Other group wants to merge with you or simply take your practice. Obamacare. What were they thinking but it doesn't really matter because you are afraid that your income is going to go down. The hospital wants to terminate your exclusive contract. Give it to the low cost guys who'll soon be employing you or not employing you — if you'll only take less.

Like that future? Many, maybe most, groups and individual physicians don't.

The real question is what are you going to do about it.

It's like you're on a track and you're headed into a tunnel and there's a train coming the other way and you can see its light shining and getting bigger and bigger and you're just a small train, like Thomas the Tank Engine and it's the Super Chief.

But real life isn't like that. You're not on a track. There are many options. There always are. It takes time to consider them. To sort out the issues. To simplify the problems. To select a strategy. To implement it. To create choices. At a minimum to create leverage in negotiations. At a maximum to create real alternatives for your success.

The alternative is to stay on that track.

That's probably where many will stay:

Freedom of choice
Is what you got
Freedom from choice
Is what you want

(Devo, Freedom of Choice, by Gerald Casale and Mark Mothersbaugh)

OPTING OUT TO OPT IN FOR YOURSELF

I'm no enemy of fast food. I just don't want to eat it. I don't care if you do. I wouldn't make it illegal. But some mayors would.

In the socialist worldview, it's all about top down control. For example, making everyone buy health insurance and then dictating what insurance companies must cover and prohibiting them from screening for preexisting conditions. Or, for example, empowering hospitals to control ACOs and dispensing with the former "logic" of anti-kickback, self-referral and antitrust laws to permit them to herd physicians into the new program.

Some, a few, physicians had already opted out of the government system (Medicare) and out of the insurance system as well, going into "concierge" medicine. They were criticized as somehow being "less than" for not wanting to be a public utility. For not wanting to be sheep.

Although many physicians are rushing into ACO models, hospital employment and other "alignment," as that system fails, not just economically but in terms of the quality of care and, importantly, the quality of experience, those with the means to do so will opt out. And that presents an opportunity for physicians entrepreneurial enough to establish practices and networks to provide what those patients want.

As the British National Health Service, and many fast food chains, prove, delivering slop is acceptable to many. But others are willing to pay top dollar for quality care and, more importantly, setting aside statistical notions of quality, for high quality wrapped in a high value qualitative experience.

I don't care how many Whoppers I can get for $5. Do you?

"CHOOSE PATIENTS OVER PROFITS" AND THE PROPAGANDA OF POLITICS

"This is a golden opportunity to choose patients over profit" said U.S. Representative Jackie Speier as she announced the "Promoting Integrity In Medicare Act of 2013," HR 2914.

In Speier's words, the bill removes Stark in-office ancillary services safe harbor protection for advanced imaging, anatomic pathology, radiation therapy and physical therapy.

I'm not in this post taking a position on changing the in-office safe harbor. Rather, let's look at the propaganda here: "Choose patients over profits"

Profits are bad. Patients are good. Completely logical if you're a Congresswoman from the San Francisco Bay Area as long as we're not talking about the tech companies in her congressional district.

But without profits, no one is going to be treating patients. So what Jackie really means, is that more profits than she thinks should be made are "bad."

What happens if what Jackie thinks is enough profit is actually not sufficient to keep doctors in the system, as in doctors dropping out of Medicare (which is happening at an increasing rate)?

Then the empress will have no clothes.
She will have chosen politics over patients.

Hmm, not a bad sound bite.

SHOCKING! NO PHYSICIAN FINANCIAL BENEFIT FROM ACO PARTICIPATION

A recent survey conducted by Jackson Healthcare reveals that sixty-seven percent of physician respondents who participated in an ACO last year reported no personal financial benefit (in the form of a bonus, shared savings arrangement, etc.) as a result of their participation. (http://www.jacksonhealthcare.com/physiciantrends2013)

Why would anybody be surprised by this result?

As I have consistently pointed out, ACOs are about shifting control and financial rewards away from physicians, in favor of hospitals and payors, that is, chiefly the government as payor via Medicare.

Creating additional levels of bureaucracy – more paperwork, more direction, more top-down control – leaves less time for patient care, at least for care that is customized as opposed to cookie cutter. It leads to physician dissatisfaction and less, not more, job security.

Physicians participating in ACOs through hospital employment or affiliation via a captive medical group or foundation must develop networks to assist them in post ACO employment. Create options and alternatives.

Medical groups participating in ACOs through provider agreements while maintaining their independent practice need to avoid ceding too much control to the ACO and must structure their operation in a way that becomes less dependent upon the failure or success of the ACO.

Healthcare business and delivery models come and go. The secret is not to become so invested in their success that their failure causes yours.

BEAN COUNTERS 1, PATIENTS 0

Japanese baseball was in a slump. With home runs down and the game seeing attendance dropping due to cited boredom, things sprang back to life this year: the number of home runs spiked and fans went wild once again.

But what was the cause of this good fortune for the league and its team owners?

After denying that their luck had anything to do with a "fixed" ball, it turned out that it had everything to do with it: League officials has instructed the official ball manufacturer to alter the ball's core to give it more "bounce" against the bat.

In the healthcare world being ushered in by Obamacare, measurement of "care" will count for more than the actual care itself.

And soon, when the measuring doesn't pan out as expected by the hospital or by the government, expect them to change what's being measured, to give the metaphorical ball a little more bounce, so to speak.

The stats will look great, the CEO will get a bonus, and no one will suffer...at least no one who counts in the new equation.

PHYSICIANS TO SUBSIDIZE SUBSIDIZED HEALTH INSURANCE EXCHANGE PARTICIPANTS

Get ready for subsidized care — I'm talking both subsidized health exchange premiums courtesy of your tax dollars, and the very real possibility that you'll be further subsidizing exchange participants' care 100% on the dollar.

Although the Affordable Care Act requires that an insurer must give three months' notice to subsidized healthcare exchange participants who fail to pay their share of premiums before the insurer can cancel coverage, the insurer has no obligation to pay for the participants' care after the first month of that three month period.

So, who pays for care if the participant doesn't reinstate his coverage on time: You do.

To complicate matters, these people will be "covered" the entire time, at least in terms of having coverage in place. However, they'll have actual coverage…the kind that you can put in the bank…only for the first month. So, you'll only learn that you'll be stuck after the fact.

In fact, it's conceivable that the carrier will pay you, only to claw the payment back after the entire three month period runs without reinstatement, due to no legal liability to have made the payment in the first place.

What's this mean for you, other than, of course, that you've become a social welfare agency?

You must review all payor contracts for the way that they impact your liability under these circumstances and renegotiate if necessary. For hospital based groups, consider ways to shift risk to the hospital as a part of your exclusive contract negotiations.

CYPRUS, USA

If you've been reading the international news, you're probably familiar with the fact that the government of Cyprus, a European Union member, is under pressure from the European Central Bank to seize funds in private depositors' bank accounts to bail out Cypriot banks.

Although when first floated, all accounts were targeted for seizure in varying percentages, the latest plan seems to include only those who were good at saving, those with more than 100,000 Euros in the bank. Up to 60% of the amount on deposit might be seized.

Imagine someone who works their whole life, saves their money and keeps it liquid in a bank account – no crazy speculation for him! – only to find that he's paying the price for the bank's foolish behavior. Depositors like him, who never stood to realize an upside in terms of distributions of the bank's profits, got only the downside via confiscation.

Upon reflection, how different is balancing a banking system failure on the heads of the productive from balancing the books of the healthcare system by reducing reimbursement to physicians? Same work. Less pay. But hey, it's patriotic.

Still complaining? Don't you know that you're just paying your fair share?

DO YOU REALLY WANT THIS SMALLER FUTURE?

In a very well written article by Cat Vasko, editor of Medical Imaging Review, *Accountable Radiology: Eliminating Sleepless Nights*, Vasko covers the comments of James Reinertsen, M.D. of the Reinertsen Group, a consultant, at a 2012 American College of Radiology conference.

In a nutshell, Reinertsen states that radiologists should reconcile themselves to lower incomes and simply focus on quality.

Although all should laud Dr. Reinertsen's comments about the need to focus on quality of care, he does a wonderful job of explaining the future of radiology, indeed, of all physicians, from the hospital and government perspective:

- You should see world as half empty.
- You will work for less.
- Suck it up, no one in the real world cares if your income drops 30%, you're still among the 1%.

Just as obviously, any radiologist who wants to be successful should see that this Reinertsen fellow's advice to settle for less is worthless, that is, unless you like the future he has planned for you.

The reason why fixed salary systems lauded by this guy drive cooperation between specialists and reduce "overuse" is that they create a perverse incentive not to work. Visit your local department of motor vehicles office and see how it plays out.

In my work with radiologists and other physician groups across the country, I often encounter this same defeatist attitude from physicians, and hear the same advice to get used to the new world of less pay from hospital administrators and their industry consultants.

Instead, assuming that your specialty is in for a 30% reduction in volume (which does not necessarily mean a 30% reduction in reimbursement), strategic group leaders need to think how to adjust staffing and how to expand their business to counter negative pressure on overall compensation.

Reinertsen is quoted as saying that the ACO is about accountability to patients. It's not: It's about accountability to the accountant types who will judge your quality based upon what's easy to measure, engage in past-based cost accounting, and award you your little slice of their pie.

Smarter medical groups leaders will instead seek to make their group's pie bigger.

It's time to get baking.

PRESERVING THE PAST

Tension, lots of tension about what to do, but that doesn't mean that always doing nothing is the right response.

It's certainly true that knowing what not to do, from individual actions to projects that could be pursued but which are passed on, is as important as taking affirmative action on those projects that will be pursued. At the same time, however, this is a very different concept from devoting close to all of your attention on preserving your current position which, really is equivalent to preserving the past.

Physician groups are under tremendous pressure, the bull's-eye of the target toward which the arrows of ACOs, hospital-centric healthcare, physician employment, Obamacare, national group competition, and more, are aimed.

What's needed is for group leaders to devote significant time to how they're going to transform their businesses to not only evade those attacks, but to capture new ground themselves.

I'm not suggesting that groups abandon their present relationships – certainly, you need to hedge more speculative ventures with a strong base. But query how strong that base really is.

Leadership And Medical Groups

SAY, DO YOUR GROUP MEMBERS HAVE THIS MINDSET?

Jean-Baptiste Say, the late-18th and early-19th Century businessman and economist, defined an entrepreneur as someone who shifts economic resources out of an area of lower and into an area of higher productivity and greater yield.

At its heart this is about creating value, value for the buyer, whether the buyer is a customer, client, patient or however described. Creating value in the context of a professional service involves delivering both an exceptional service and an exceptional experience. The mindset of an entrepreneur is tuned to deliver accordingly.

Distinguish this from the mindset of a bureaucrat – someone who goes about his or her tasks just following the rules but not creating anything of value.

No matter how much attention you, as a group leader, may have devoted to developing an Experience Monopoly™ for your group's customers, the facilities, referral sources and patients, if your group's members lack an entrepreneurial drive, the chances are great that although there may be delivering good care, that's all they're delivering.

How would you describe the mindset of the members of your group?

Are they simply delivering medical care at, or even above, the level of the community standard? No negligence there, but no delight created, either.

WHAT'S YOUR HIGHEST AND BEST USE?

What's the highest and best use of your time as a medical group leader?

Is it devoting time to your group's business and its future or is it delivering patient care?

Any one of your group's members should excel in terms of patient care – that's one of the reasons, yes, just one of the reasons, you hired them.

But very few of them could perform the role of group leader. That's what you are supposed to be doing.

So, why aren't you allocating your time to leadership?

It might be your choice to do otherwise, or it might be the only option available to you as a result of the group's choice.

Either way, its not your highest and best use and it's not the group's either.

MASTERY AND YOUR MEDICAL GROUP

I'm not really one for documentaries, but I recently watched, for the second time, Jiro Dreams of Sushi.

Facially about an octogenarian's lifelong quest to serve the best sushi possible, it's true lesson is the role of mastery, the continuous path of excellence in an endeavor.

Physicians, no, all professionals, should be on a similar route to continuous improvement.

But for medical group leaders, the real question in both hiring and retaining physicians is what is within the scope of mastery.

Clearly, mastery in patient care, while absolutely required, is no longer sufficient. Physicians seeking only medical mastery will not advance your group's interests. The scope of the quest must be broader.

Think of an airline flight from Los Angeles to Chicago. The mastery of the pilots, who even after flying for decades are still involved in training and improvement, got you to the destination safely and on time. Yet often the overall experience falls short, from the hassles of boarding to delayed or lost luggage.

Mastery for medical groups, like for airlines or my own services, must broaden to cover the entire customer experience.

The process for your group starts with hiring the right people, people who are on this quest. Then, your employment agreements or independent contractor agreements and the group's compensation plan and rules and regulations must all support and incentivize this broader notion of mastery. And, you must continue to train and reinforce the group's expectations.

Years ago, many, many years ago, I had surgery on my wrist. Almost miraculously, from a lay perspective, I was "cured." Yet to this day, I vividly recall the hand surgeon's complete lack of personality and the anesthesiologist screaming at his divorce lawyer over the phone in both pre-op and post-op. True masters of their craft? Each would say "yes" and so too might their certifying Boards. But would I ever recommend them? Hardly.

In today's market, as medicine becomes more commoditized, as referral and exclusive contract relationships are destabilized, overall mastery is more important than ever in distinguishing what your group provides, in creating an Experience Monopoly™ — an experience for your patients, referral sources and facilities that they cannot get from anyone else.

People fly from around the world to have dinner at Jiro's, paying around $300 for 15 or so pieces of sushi. His fish aren't swimming in the sea of "good enough," and neither should yours.

WHY DOCUMENT THE VALUE OF A GROUP MEMBER'S INTEREST?

They say that beauty is in the eyes of the beholder.

But the value of a physician's interest in a medical group is in the eyes of the holder — the holder of the pen, so to speak: those in control of the terms of the buy-in and buy-out provisions of your group's shareholders or partnership agreement.

So what's a membership interest worth?

No time to think about this now? Fine with me.

But it's not going to be fine for you because sooner rather than later someone is going to leave the group and they are going to demand "their share."

They'll claim that the group really doesn't exist – it was just a pass through and they want their accounts receivable. Or worse, they'll claim the group and you, yes, you, personally, owe them a fiduciary duty to schedule them and to collect "their" accounts receivable. "So where's my money!"

What is the formula for determining value? Does that formula trigger or destroy other rights and privileges that the group wants to assert in its organizational documents?

Think about it. Now.

It's better than worrying about it, or being sued, later.

I WENT TO A FOOD FAIR. CAN REFERRAL SOURCES FIND YOU?

I went to a food fair. You know, one of those "Taste of Fill-In-The Blank" fairs where restaurants of all sorts sell sample size versions of their food.

The whole idea for the restaurants is to get people interested in coming to their real place. They are never going to make any real money selling samples for $3.

Most of the restaurants sold their samples from booths. A few had fancy trailers with their names emblazoned on them. But the booths were really plain, like the kind at an elementary school fair that sells hot dogs or at which you lob a ping pong ball to try to get it into a fishbowl to win a goldfish. (It might not be PC to do that anymore but you are probably old enough to remember back to when it was OK to think the way you wanted to.)

Anyway, these restaurants must have paid a lot to rent space at the "Taste of" and in some cases they probably didn't make much or any profit at the $3 price tag. But what hit me is that while the booths had the restaurants' names on them, only a handful of them out of probably a hundred had their address. Good food? Check. Smiling faces? Check. Want to actually go to their restaurant and pay more for a whole lunch or dinner? Check. But where in heck are they located??!!

What are you doing to let people know where to find you?

You're probably not doing doctoring at the local "Taste of" or even at a health fair, but what I mean is what are you doing so that potential new facilities or potential new referral sources or potential new patients can find out about you and where you are located? Even if you're an employee of some hospital or large medical group, how can potential other employers find out about you?

What are you doing to advertise your fare?

Right now, it's time for dinner. I had a really great lamb in pita sandwich at the fair. Was it a Greek restaurant stand? Or maybe it was Turkish? I know I might be able to find it. Or not. I guess I'll just go to have pizza down the street. I know where that place is.

IS YOUR GROUP A SLOW LORIS OR A SITTING DUCK?

Years ago, the Santa Barbara Zoo had a fascinating animal on display, a slow loris.

A type of primate, the rainforest creature evades predators by moving very, very, very slowly. In fact, even slower than that. Its predators spot prey as a result of movement – the slow loris almost stands still while moving.

Unlike slow lorises, glacial speed is not a medical group's friend. Your predators have an easier time spotting your weaknesses when you're standing still. Your leaders gain nothing by simply protecting the status quo.

Stop thinking of slow lorises and start thinking about ducks, sitting ducks, that is.

"We've held the contract for 20 years."

"The Jones Group always sends their referrals to us."

"Bob went to boarding school with the CEO; we're in a protected position."

In an isolated sense, there's truth in each of those statements and there's nothing inherently wrong with reciting them.

But in connection with the functioning of the many interrelated systems in which these relationships exist, they are not determinative.

As Peter Drucker said, ""Because the purpose of business is to create a customer, the business enterprise has two–and only two–basic functions: marketing and innovation."

Going beyond that point, the goal is to retain the customer, have him, her or it buy more of your services, all while you are marketing to other potential customers and creating new "circles."

But without change through innovation, without expansion of your service offerings, you become close to calcified. And while that's safety for slow lorises, it's the kiss of death for medical groups.

IS YOUR GROUP RUNNING ON AUTOPILOT?

I read a quote from the owner of a private boat rescue service, sort of like a floating Auto Club, who said that they have a rule of thumb: the boats with the most electronics are those most likely to run aground. That's because those boat owners place so much faith in the electronic reports of location and depth that they fail to actually look where they're going.

A similar situation affects medical groups.

Take, for example, a medical group that receives comprehensive billing service reports replete with dashboards illustrating all types of practice metrics. All appears to be not just OK, but glowingly wonderful: The group is on the right course.

But those reports may or may not be correct. And, even if they are true, they can only provide a partial picture of the group's business world, because they do not contain all of the essential information necessary to lead the group.

Consider the case of a hospital-based medical group that is in trouble. Dissatisfaction among the rank and file over the assignment of cases and the amount of compensation leads to an eruption over leadership. The hospital is on the group's case, pressing for a major change in structure:

bring more "fairness" to the group, make everyone a partner, and perhaps do a national search for new leadership.

But the group's leaders say that the "dashboard" indicates that everything is okay.

My unfortunate observation is this this type of problem, in varying costume, is far too common.

Group leaders, and sometimes all group members, are seduced by reports that they perhaps don't understand or which perhaps don't actually make sense or report the truth, or they place all of their faith on reports which are highly accurate but which contain no data on matters outside the scope of those reports – such as issues involving compensation, the relationship between group physicians and hospital staff, and issues of importance to referring physicians and patients.

Just as on the sea, the data that's collected and reported is of value, but you've got to keep your eyes open as well.

DOES YOUR MEDICAL GROUP SUFFER FROM THIS COMMON TRAGEDY?

In economic and ecological terms, the "tragedy of the commons" describes a situation in which those participating in a shared or common benefit, such as grazing rights on a traditional British or American colonial "commons," abuse the fact that they are each entitled to the benefit of use but bear only a proportionate share of the upkeep or downside.

The same concept also applies to professional firms such as medical groups.

Each member seeks to engage in more of the activity that is directly and temporally tied to increasing his or her income, such as generating more compensable work units or minutes. On the other hand, there is no immediately obvious benefit from time and effort spent on group strategy, policy, management and other long-term issues. Each participant considers that someone else's job — someone else will take care of that.

Just as the traditional British commons suffered from overuse and under-care, so, too, does a medical group's fate suffer from the failure of its members to devote the proper care to its longer-term future.

Solutions to avoid the tragedy include establishing proper group governance structures, selecting the right leaders who are not only charged with the power to lead but with the ability to make decisions as well, and establishing compensation systems that reward for time devoted to not simply day to day management but to charting the group's course into the future, as well.

A KODAK MOMENT

I remember, as a kid, walking around Disneyland, noticing yellow "no parking" size signs labeled Kodak Moment. They indicated a great vantage point for taking a photo.

When Kodak was challenged by Fuji for dominance in the sale of photographic film, Kodak succeeded by changing the value proposition. They were no longer in the photo business, they were in the memory business. And who better to protect your memories, the cheaper alternative, Fuji, or the company synonymous with photography, Kodak? The answer was obvious.

Yet today Kodak is in bankruptcy, its core film business gutted by the digital camera.

What's darkly funny about this is that Kodak invented digital photography, yet chose largely to ignore it. Perhaps Kodak was too large to truly innovate. Perhaps it was too focused on film to make the switch to digital. Perhaps its employees, from executives to those working in its manufacturing plants, were economically handcuffed to film photography.

The same phenomenon is common in healthcare.

Many medical groups, especially hospital-based medical groups, choose, sometimes intentionally and sometimes simply by default, to ignore the fact that unless they establish an identity separate and apart from hospitals, their businesses will soon be obsolete.

Of course, their medical specialty will likely continue – but it will be controlled by someone else, whether by hospitals or by large groups which disrupt their business relationships.

Start taking action now to avoid having your own Kodak Moment.

DOES YOUR GROUP BELIEVE IN ITSELF?

Too many medical groups simply don't believe in themselves.

How else could you explain why a group leader would spend $600 on dinner but not $300,000 to preserve the group's $20,000,000 a year business?

The first offers little to no ROI (it does provide a few hours of satisfaction and some nutrients) while the other would yield a 6,500% return over first year alone. Try getting that at the bank.

It's not the price tag. Depending on the medical specialty, the $20,000,000 a year group devotes well over $300,000 to many categories on the expense-side.

Perhaps it's the naive belief that the group's business will simply continue, year after year, like some perpetual motion machine, powered only by the first push.

Or perhaps it's the failure to realize that not devoting the proper resources to your future is the far more expensive alternative.

NO MORE ROOM FOR AVERAGE

There's no more room for average in terms of any medical practice's business approach. This applies regardless of specialty or whether you are hospital-based or office-based. This applies whether you are in solo practice or with a group.

Medical practice is becoming stratified. Some practices are aligning with ACO's. Some practices are taking action to go a completely independent route. Some practices are merging or forming other alignment with other practices as opposed to with hospitals. Some practices are opting out of government financed care completely.

In some instances in life and in business, it pays to wait and see. In other instances, after weighing alternatives, it pays to do nothing. But this is neither of those instances.

Rather, not taking any action puts your practice into a position equivalent to that of a ship dead in the water.

It's obvious that the current system is broken – no matter who you think broke it.

Doing nothing is not the cure.

Wait and see is what got you into this mess.

Set a strategy for your group's future and implement it. Note that unlike a ship, your group can hedge its bets and adopt more than one strategy – that is not the same as doing nothing.

MEDICAL GROUPS' TWO MAJOR PROBLEMS

I see two very common problems with medical groups.

They move too slow.

They do what everyone else does.

In this market – a still-sick economy, the push toward ACOs and other so-called "alignment," and the other ills of Obamacare – many are pushing toward becoming large. But large makes them fragile — prone to eventual failure — they just don't realize it.

Instead, you want to develop speed — speed in making decisions, speed in setting strategy, speed in adjusting strategy, speed in implementing tactics.

Too much hassle? Just want to treat patients? Then just close up your practice and go get a job.

Look, the end game is going to be won through speed and innovation, not size.

Sure, almost everyone else is going to say you're wrong, that that's not what everyone else is doing.

But that's why they're average — they are doing what everyone else is doing.

You need to take a hammer to average.

MERGERS: PAUSE AND QUESTION

Strength in numbers. Or is there?

Medical groups seeking alternatives to the sale of their practice to a hospital often consider merging with another group.

There's nothing wrong with the notion of a merger. Often, there's something right. But not always.

For example, merging two weak performing groups rarely creates a strong one. Think Sears plus Kmart.

Merging even two strong groups can be problematic, as there's far more to a successful merger than balance sheets — focus, personnel, management style and group culture play determinative roles.

I'm not saying don't consider a merger: If you're looking at alternatives you have to. But seek the **right** merger partner — a strategic merger, one in which one plus one equals 3 or more. Bad math, but good business.

IT'S NEVER THE RIGHT TIME SO IT'S ALWAYS THE RIGHT TIME

I'm too busy right now.

There's too much going on.

Mañana.

Maybe next year.

Medical group leaders are busy focusing on day to day activities: Most are deeply involved in direct patient care. Some, yes, some, also devote some time to working on their business.

But there's a pressing need to engage in strategy. And you have to address the tough issues, like governance, succession planning, compliance, expansion of your business, and many more.

Yes, you're right, it's not the right time. In fact, it's **never** the right time.

So if there's never a right time but you have to take action anyway, then consider that it's always the right time.

Get started. Because one thing's for sure. The "unexpected" really isn't and it's better to be prepared.

WHY YOU SHOULDN'T WASTE YOUR MONEY HOLDING A "STRATEGIC PLANNING" RETREAT

Here's something you can absolutely plan on: most planning done by medical groups, especially that common variety, the "strategic planning retreat," is a complete waste of time.

Determining strategy has nothing to do with planning. Planning is a process of projecting from the present, while strategy is the opposite: it's selecting a desired future from among alternatives, which future is then harnessed to pull you toward it.

Developing strategy only starts at a meeting such as a retreat: that's simply a step in a complete, larger, ongoing process.

Sure, spending $10,000 or $20,000 to facilitate a "planning retreat" is far less than the investment required to develop a true strategy, but the reality is that it's $10,000 or $20,000 wasted.

Let's get strategic.

MISTAKES HAPPEN

Mistakes happen.

There's a divergence of opinion on the question of whether or not to apologize or express sorrow over a healthcare error.

Will it lead to increased chances of malpractice litigation and be construed as an admission of liability? Thirty-six states, including California and Texas, have enacted laws protecting certain expressions of sorry and remorse from being admissible in court.

Recently, I was on an American Airlines flight. A flight attendant carrying a tray with a filled red wine glass lost her balance and dumped the wine on my shoulder, down my back and onto, well, my, err, seat. She immediately and profusely apologized and said that she'd get me a cleaning voucher. I smiled and told her that it was OK. She told me that most passengers would have screamed at her or threatened to get her fired.

Mistakes happen, and it's often how the mistake maker, not the "victim," reacts that makes the difference in the outcome.

If your state immunizes apologies, does your group have a policy on when, how and what to say? Let's talk about it.

TRANSPARENCY WITHIN MEDICAL GROUPS

Secrecy. Data gathering. Keeping safe from those who want to do you harm.

Hot topics in the news as I write this. But I'm not writing from a political point of view. At least not this time.

Instead, I'm writing about protecting your medical group's financial and performance data and about guarding its yet unfolded strategies.

In particular, I'm writing about the question of how much transparency should exist within your group.

The answer requires a particular balance, one that must be determined on a group by group basis: there is no hard and fast rule.

However, keep in mind that the most successful groups, the Strategic Groups™, are not run as clubs. They are not completely transparent.

On the other hand, sharing some amount of performance data across the entire group, whether you see that as only owner physicians, or as all providers, can be a tremendous motivator in the development of a cohesive team.

But pure matters of strategy and your group's essential financial information should be held much closer to the vest. Those entrusted with it should be bound by fiduciary duty and by confidentiality agreements. Unfortunately, any of your inner circle might be tomorrow's competitor.

There is no advantage to be gained in claiming to be the most transparent while actually being anything but. There's also no advantage to disclosing willy-nilly what should be protected information. Instead, find the right balance for your group and clearly establish walls beyond which information is closely guarded against attack both from outside and from inside your group.

ARE SOME PARTNERS LESS EQUAL BUT JUST AS LIABLE?

Many medical groups operate as partnerships, generally partnerships of professional corporations. The reason for that structure is simple: it allows maximum flexibility in terms of each owner's management of his or her related business and tax attributes, while preserving a high degree of protection from liability.

Note that I said "a high degree" because there is never a situation in which there can be total protection from liability.

At the same time, many groups have compensation plans that reward different partners, or different classes of partners, differently, such that there is a spread, sometimes a wide spread, in compensation.

One complication of this type structure is that while all partners are jointly and severally liable for the debts of the partnership, some partners are reaping a much greater financial reward. And, in some instances, that reward is not tied to the fact that they are devoting more time, or harder effort, or even smarter effort to the venture.

In some cases, this situation is intended and understood by all. But in others, it is a situation arrived at blindly.

When did you last look at your partnership agreement? Does it create the liability result that was intended?

IS THERE THIS DISCONNECT WITHIN YOUR MEDICAL GROUP?

If you want to go to the movies but your spouse wants to go to a play, you've reached an impasse. But that's simply a minor issue, one that can, of course, grow.

But if you always want to go to the movies and your spouse never does, while your spouse always wants to go to plays but you never do, then you have a much bigger problem.

Now shift this over to any business organization, in your case, probably your medical group. The same dynamic appears when one partner or one set of partners wants to move the business in one direction while the others want to go in another, or even more likely, don't want to go in any direction at all.

If this were your weekend basketball team, you'd be concerned.

It's your life, treat is as seriously.

Consider a twenty-some person medical group with polarized groups of members. At one end of the spectrum, some of the owners want to expand the group to other sites and to aggressively compete for new business. At the other end, no one wants to expend a cent — just keep the distributions to the owners as high as possible.

We all know that there are tectonic shifts impacting the healthcare industry. If your group can't develop a strategy for its future because of internal dissension, then, by default, you're allowing someone else — the hospital, the government, your competitors — to choose a future for you. (It won't be very pretty.)

Resolve the impasse or resolve to choose another career path, because this one's a dead end.

NO MEETING OF THE MINDS

Is your medical group slowing down success, wasting time in management meetings?

Imagine a group that holds a meeting of its bloated board each week. Over a dozen people sit at the table, each putting in his three or four cents worth, even when he or she has so sense. Protecting fiefdoms. Feigning expertise. Micromanaging. (Micromanagement by an individual is bad enough, but micromanagement by committee is sheer hell.)

Sure, there are a few legitimate reasons for groups to have leadership meetings, whether face to face or electronically, such as when you need to pull together a number of ideas to plan a new initiative.

But the majority of meetings, those devoted to exchanging information, are a pure waste of time. Send a memo. Send an email. Or even a note by carrier pigeon. But don't waste time and meet.

Sure, business decisions require some thinking. But the question is who should be doing the thinking, and the answer is as few people as possible.

And, those people, those leaders of your group, must be empowered to make decisions – that is, empowered to lead. It doesn't matter whether your leaders are elected or chosen as a result of the drawing the short stick. Heck, just throw a dart at a list of your group's owners and anoint the holey one as the leader. Any of those is better than management by committee.

TECHNOLOGY, RULES AND COMPLIANCE

Technology is neither inherently good nor inherently bad. It's good only if it does something beneficial – makes things faster, easier, cheaper, or better. And then, of course, the question is faster, easier, cheaper or better for whom?

I recently went with my son to a trendy burger place in Westwood, adjacent to UCLA. For an upscale fast food place, the interior design was top-notch. However, as opposed to ordering from an employee at the counter, you're directed to one of two iPads mounted on the wall, each mated with a credit card reader.

Very trendy, but very slow. First you build your burger, then you order fries, then you order a drink — one at a time. We moved through the process as quickly as it allowed, but it took at least 4 minutes from start to finish.

Because we beat the lunch crowd, and had only a few minutes wait to use the iPad, the time spent was not much of a problem. However, within a few minutes there was a line out the door.

Yes, the technology certainly looked trendy. It enabled the restaurant to have one employee at the counter to monitor things and deliver the food, as opposed to having a larger payroll. However, if I had to stand in a long line to wait for an iPad to open up, I'd probably go someplace else.

It occurs to me that the indiscriminate use of technology, or the use of it to benefit the wrong party, is akin to the adoption and enforcement of rules.

Take, for example, a rule requiring the completion of a certain form in your practice that duplicates information captured elsewhere. Perhaps it's a form required of patients. Perhaps it's a form required of your group's physicians. For whose benefit was the rule adopted? How can it be made to also benefit the person having to comply? What incentives can be tied to compliance?

What the burger place thought was cool technology that reduced their labor costs was, from the customer's perspective, a pain in the ass. It would've taken 45 seconds to place the order with a live person as opposed to 4 minutes with the machine. And, the restaurant completely overlooked the notion of programming any attempt to up-sell the order – "Would you like fries with that?"

Are your group's rules built from the same stuff? Are the hospital's?

When you have trouble with compliance, think about it from that perspective.

Negotiation & Contracting

AN EXCLUSIVE CONTRACT RENEWAL CHOICE: NO THANK YOU

Hospital based medical groups are often faced with a choice upon exclusive contract renewal: The expectation or demand on the part of the hospital that the group must provide its services, perhaps even at a higher level of intensity, for lower or no stipend support.

A group enters into an exclusive contract in order to protect its turf. In return, it takes on the obligation to provide coverage. But if, without stipend support from the hospital at an acceptable level, the group cannot recruit and retain its providers, then, if we assume that its billing and collections have already been maximized, the group has only a few choices if it wishes to remain committed to the obligation to provide coverage:

1. It can negotiate a more efficient coverage schedule.
2. It can reduce compensation to its existing providers.
3. It can attempt to find new providers willing to work for less.
4. If applicable in the medical specialty, it can shift work to allied healthcare professionals.

Alternatively, and usually not considered, the group can choose not to renew the contract. If the group had adopted a business-like attitude, it will have already expanded its business to other facilities. If it hadn't expanded, the choices are closing up shop — there'd be no reason to exist — or to attempt to continue to provide services at the facility on a request only basis, perhaps with a pared down staff.

Most group leaders will probably consider that last option unworkable. But query whether, with more hospitals pushing for lower to no stipends, and with regional groups having the power to walk away from unprofitable deals, whether more hospitals will be left begging for any assistance at all from hospital-based specialists?

TRUST BUT VERIFY

You're the leader of a medical group. One of your group's employees, Dr. Bob, wants to borrow $10,000. He's worked with the group for eight years, and you know him well. He's trustworthy.

Bob promises to pay the group back in three months.

Do you simply write a Bob a check or do get him to sign a promissory note?

"Trust but verify," Ronald Reagan's maxim when dealing with the Soviet Union, would certainly apply. You'd get the note.

Now let's switch gears. You're not dealing with Dr. Bob about a short term loan, you're in the throes of the negotiation over a contract with the hospital's CEO. Let's call him Robert.

You've known Robert for years. He's always been true to his word.

You negotiate for a provision, for example, a cost of living increase to be applied to a coverage stipend. Robert says he'll take are of it, you have his word, but he just doesn't want to put it into the contract. Then he adds, "you can trust me."

No matter your personal relationship with Robert, no matter the years of history, you must apply the same Reagan Rule – verify by way of putting the verbal promises into the agreement.

Even if you completely trust Robert, you don't know if the hospital board is going to pressure him to do something that he doesn't personally agree with, you don't know whether he'll even be the CEO a month from now, and you can never rely on the bond of "business friendship."

Trust, but verify.

TERMINATION NOTICE

"Bob, we've got to give you your two weeks notice. Here's a check for the next two weeks' compensation. Just pack your personal belongings and Jerry, here, will see you to the door."

Of course, if your medical group has a contract with a facility, say an exclusive contract, it can't technically be "fired." But its contract can be "terminated." If there's a without cause termination provision, especially a short one, in the contract, it might be a distinction without a difference. You'll still be looking for a new job.

In times like these, when larger groups are displacing local ones with greater frequency and the power is shifting in favor of facilities and away from physicians, it's time to rethink agreeing to short without cause termination provisions.

First, especially if you've ignored my argument that it's essential that your group provide services at multiple facilities to create a safety net against over-reliance on one facility relationship, 90 days if not nearly enough notice to either find another "home" or wind up doing business and find your group's members other jobs.

Second, depending on your state's laws, the 90 day termination notice period might be a cap on the length of contract damages in the event the facility simply tosses you out without notice or otherwise breaches your agreement.

Termination provisions and provisions governing what happens upon termination are taking on larger importance in any medical group deal.

CONTRACTS DON'T CONTAIN EXTRA BAGGAGE

Imagine that you are an engineer packing a space vehicle for flight. You'd include what you'd intend be used and toss in some backups – but you certainly wouldn't include anything that won't be required.

The same rule holds true with provisions in contracts, from seemingly simple employment agreements to inch-plus thick exclusive contracts.

No matter what the other negotiator says, no matter how lovingly she explains that section such-and-such is simply "corporate policy," and no matter how wonderful your relationship with her ("She'd never screw the group over, we've known her for years!"), each provision in an agreement is a tool that's intended to be used.

For your safety, consider the phrase "intended to be used" as including "against you." Just as in packing for a space flight, there is no extra baggage in that contract.

LOOK BEFORE YOU LEAP: DOCUMENT YOUR DEAL

1. Look before you leap. CHECK.

2. Measure twice, cut once. CHECK.

3. Document your deal with your partners before commencing joint practice. WHAT?

As simple as it seems, many disputes between physicians, from office sharing deals gone wrong, to full on disputes over the compensation from a practice partnership, occur because no one bothered to work out the details and preserve them in a contact before the deal began.

Yes, only three steps: 1. Plan it out. 2. Memorialize the deal. 3. Do steps 1 and 2 before starting the business of the venture.

"But it takes time!" "But it costs money." Yes and yes. But the effort and investment involved pale in comparison to the effort and investment you will devote to the dispute that will follow if you don't make the effort and the investment ahead of time.

100% AIR CONDITIONED

The old hotel stood on a corner 10 or 15 blocks from the new center of downtown, run-down curtains visible through the windows of its 10 story dirty brick hulk. But it was the red neon sign, with letters at least 5 feet high stretched all the way across the building just beneath the roof line that caught my attention: "100% Air Conditioned."

At the time the building was built, my guess is the 1930's, a completely air-conditioned hotel was an incredible competitive advantage. I imagine that guests flocked to it, ready to plunk down cash – this was way before credit cards – to do business with the hotel. But today, air conditioning is not even a question on the minds of potential guests.

It's not much different when it comes to the question of a medical group's competitive advantage in attracting contracting partners. Do you have one?

Competitive advantages are developed, excluding competitors from the equation. But as soon as one's competitors catch up, what was once an advantage becomes simply the price of admission.

Negotiating a contract and properly documenting it are important functions, but they can only take place in a larger context, the context being a decision by the parties to do business together. The advantage your group offers a prospective contracting partner is the glue that binds.

So what exactly is your group's competitive advantage? Does it have one? Have you revisited it and updated for the current market? Or, is it something akin to "100% air-conditioned?"

What do you think?

FALSE POSITIVES AND MEDICAL GROUP LEADERSHIP

False positives. A significant problem in medicine.

And I'm not even talking about diagnostic tests, I am talking about the indicators that many physicians believe demonstrate leadership ability.

Consider a physician who is seen as "tough" in connection with business.

"We should demand an increase in our stipend from the hospital!"

"We are paying our employees too much!"

"We need to negotiate a lower rate with our billing service!"

Yet the same physician habitually shows up late for work, launches into rants, complains to referral sources, and generally pisses people off left and right.

Toughness is not itself good business sense. It is itself not leadership. Yet many believe it to be a positive trait.

On its own, in context, toughness may be a trait of leaders, at least of some leaders, but it is not a determinative trait and it certainly is not leadership or business acumen in and of itself.

It can also be the trait of a jerk. Of someone who will destroy your group, its relationships and its practice.

DON'T FALL IN LOVE WITH ANY ONE DEAL

Your house is for sale.

A potential buyer comes along. You are happy. You let the buyer know that you'd love to sell to him. You don't look for other offers.

Ridiculous, you say?

Yes, I agree, you'd never do that with your house, but physicians do it all the time with their practices.

Don't fall in love with any one deal.

Find alternatives.

Don't signal neediness.

Find a strategic buyer.

Perhaps think of it this way: Your practice's house is for sale. You don't have to move.

ACOS AND NEGOTIATION

As healthcare becomes more concentrated, more hospital-centric, physicians should begin to question what rights and economic control they are ceding to the ACO or other hospital vehicle.

Many physicians believe that they have little to no negotiating power and if they believe that, it's certainly true.

But if that's the case, there'd never be negotiations in respect of an employment agreement (there is) and there'd never be negotiations in respect of an exclusive contract (there is).

So, it's really an issue of what Henry Ford stated: If you believe you can, you're right. If you believe you can't, you're right.

How right are you?

ARE YOU SELLING CHEVYS?

If you're like most people, you hate shopping for a car. But even if you hate it, you probably follow the rule of negotiating with multiple dealers. You know that you have to have alternatives to any one deal.

If you haven't already, read my post, My Father Loved To Buy Cars. And Your Exclusive Contract Or Employment Agreement, about why most medical groups don't apply the same lesson to protect and expand their businesses.

Of course, if you're selling cars, the story is different. Years ago I represented some car dealers.

Unfortunately, there's growing similarity between selling cars and selling medical care. You wish it weren't true, but wishing alone isn't going to change anything.

For car dealers, it's about distinguishing your service so that the car isn't a commodity. Or it's about creating a car that is so unique or at least so hard to find that its not that much of a commodity.

Take that to heart whether you're running a 3 doctor group or a 300 doctor group. Or even if you are an employed doctor, say one working for a hospital system.

If you are the commodity doctor, then the hospital or group will treat you as such. Let's look at the MGMA compensation survey numbers and plop you down at the median or maybe a bit more. A little bit more, but never a lot.

But if you've pushed your professional development and your referral base and your reputation beyond the tough but pervious ceiling of commodity status, hospitals might scramble to build you a "Dr. You Institute." Or you could tell them to buzz off and do it yourself.

If you're selling Chevys and Joe Customer walks in the door to buy a new Suburban, you've got to compete on price and customer service. If you're selling Ferraris, and Joe Customer walks in the door you aren't even interested in talking to him about a new car because you only sell those to existing customers — the factory doesn't even make a new car until you have it sold.

I'm not saying you can't make it up on volume if you're a commodity selling Chevy dealer. I'm saying that it's near impossible to make it up on volume as a commodity selling doctor.

Are you a Chevy dealer or a doctor?

MY FATHER LOVED TO BUY CARS. AND YOUR EXCLUSIVE CONTRACT OR EMPLOYMENT AGREEMENT.

My father loved to buy cars. Not lots of them. He wasn't a collector. I mean that he loved, really loved negotiating with car dealers. And in a way, he did buy a lot of them because back then they only lasted about 3 years, max. It seems as if he was always taking me to a car dealer. It was fun.

But my father had rules for negotiating and one of them was to always, always have an alternative. So he negotiated with multiple dealers for that white over maroon 1962 Ford Galaxie 500.

If you're like most people, you hate shopping for a car. But even if you hate it, you probably follow the rule of negotiating with multiple dealers. You know that you have to have alternatives to any one deal.

So why do you throw the rule out the window in connection with your professional practice, especially if you're a hospital-based physician group leader? Have you fallen for the lie that you are in a service relationship to Community Memorial St. Marks or whatever the name of the hospital is? Or, you think that they love you? They don't. Or, maybe they do, but their love isn't stronger than the fact that sooner or later a competitor will say that they can do it without stipend support or that they can do it better because they won some award that no one in their right mind really cares about.

So, how many alternative deals do you have in place right now for your group or for your employment contract? How many other deals are you pursuing right now?

My father loved to simply walk off the lot, leaving the deal in the air. "No," he'd say to the salesman, "you really don't want to sell a car today." And off we'd go. Usually to get ice cream.

Can you say "no" to the hospital's "final offer" because you have another deal in place? Can you just walk away and go get ice cream?

NEGOTIATION: WHY TIMES 5

There's an old negotiating story about two sisters arguing (negotiating) over the one remaining orange in the house. Each one wants it and is not willing to split it in half.

The moral of the story, and the point of this post, is the importance of the question, "Why?" So, in the orange negotiation, "Why do you want it?"

It turns out that in the case of the two sisters, one wanted the zest for a recipe and the other wanted the juice. For those unfamiliar with oranges, this means that they both could have received exactly what they wanted: A de-zested (zestless?) orange still has all of its juice.

Most negotiation in real life isn't that simple, and (unfortunately for those who spent money on the book by the title) it's generally not win-win.

But that doesn't lessen the importance of the simple question, "Why?," in negotiation. In fact, I suggest that you use the rule of "Why times 5," asking and re-asking to drill down until you can identify what your negotiating opponent is really after – it is usually not facially apparent. Once you know the real "why," it's much easier to offer a real solution, one that's perhaps totally acceptable to you.

Of course, it doesn't have to be 5 "whys," it can be 12. Or, it can be 3. The point is to ask.

For example, in a negotiation, the opposing side demanded a fixed payment in respect of licensing a product they had developed. We wanted to pay a percentage based on sales. Why did they want the fixed price? "Because it's easier?" Why is it easier? "There's no accounting involved?" Why is accounting a problem? "It takes time and effort." We then offered a transparent reporting system with open access and agreed to bear the price of monitoring. They accepted and we got our percentage deal.

Have trouble getting this? Why?

SURVEY YOURSELF

Hospitals often use surveys as a weapon to attack hospital-based groups. No matter who runs the survey, they are prone to error, misuse and out right abuse.

In fact over the last three decades, I've never seen a medical staff survey that wasn't defective. Querying all of the psychiatrists on staff about the quality of the anesthesia department is, well, crazy.

But, since hospitals love surveys, they are a good tool for you to start sponsoring yourself. Query your patients, query referring physicians and even query hospital staff.

Of course, the survey has to be designed properly. Consider also that the scope of the questions doesn't have to relate simply to the services provided by your group – it might also inquire as to the level of services provided by other physicians and by the hospital itself.

The beauty of this type of survey is that you control whether the results are released. It's a bit like creating evidence, only favorable evidence, to support your case.

WOULD YOU SIGN THIS?

"Sign this please. Right there. Yeah, there, on the last line. Next to the date."

How many times have you heard this? Ten? Twenty? Eighteen Hundred Fifty Three?

Have you always signed?

What did you get for doing so? That "what you got" is, in legal terms, the consideration for your promise. It's one of the required elements of a contract. Required in the sense of making it enforceable. No consideration, no contract.

Of course, not all of those pieces of paper shoved in front of you were contracts. Like that traffic ticket. But don't focus on that because this is not a law school class and this is not really about the legal enforceability of contacts.

Think about this as an English lesson. I want you to remember that, for you, your career, and your business, the word consideration starts with a "Why?"

As in, "why should I sign it?" What are you getting in return?

Think about this as a negotiation lesson.

The hospital administrator presents a letter to you reading that despite the scope of your exclusive contract, Dr. X will be allowed to practice in the department.

Or, the founder of a venture that you're an owner of asks you to sign an investment-related form dated five years previous, just prior to the date of your investment.

Or, you've agreed on a price, but the other side now adds a new provision. What do you get in return?

Yes, you caught me. This is really about mindset, your mindset in negotiating. In realizing that many situations are negotiations.

You don't always have to get something back, but at least think, for a moment, of what you are getting in return before you sign, or before you tell yourself that you already agreed on price so that some additional issue is just another point that they're extracting.

EMOTIONS AS DRIVERS OF CONTRACTUAL RELATIONSHIPS

I recently read in a magazine aimed at the hospital administrator market that administrators make the decision to terminate their facility's relationship with a physician group because it makes business sense to do so, and that emotion is not a part of the equation.

Although I have certainly met many hospital administrators who had no personality, or at least no readily ascertainable redeeming characteristics, they were still, to the best of my knowledge, people.

And people can't separate emotions from decision-making. They can lie about it and claim emotions are not a factor, but it's frankly impossible for emotions not to be a major driver of decision-making.

The lesson here is not that physician groups can ignore the quality of their service, including the quality of responsiveness to a hospital administration's issues. That would be foolish.

But it would be equally foolish to believe that strategies based on emotion have little value when in fact behavioral economists and psychologists who study decision-making clearly acknowledge how irrational our emotion laden decision-making it really is.

Knowing how to develop emotion-based strategies and how to implement them are simply among the "combined arms" tools that medical groups must develop in order to thrive.

RETAIN THE RIGHT TO REPURCHASE YOUR PRACTICE

You decided to sell your medical group to a large national group or to the hospital.

If you've been paying attention to my blog posts, you know that I strongly believe that the creation of large players in healthcare, especially large hospital-centric players, is making the industry far more fragile, far more prone to fail and to fail big. With size comes complexity and little, if any true economies of scale. When, not if, the economic squeeze is put on these entities, they will explode like a supernova, throwing hundreds if not thousands of physicians economically down the drain.

So, before boarding the Titanic medical group, make sure that you pack a lifeboat: negotiate to retain the right to repurchase your practice.

When the time comes, you may not want to repurchase it – there may be no value in it. But having the right to do so places you at a tremendous advantage in terms of controlling some of the downside.

Psychology of Success

EIGHTEEN WHEELERS AND THE MEDICAL GROUP ACQUISITION MEME

Eighteen wheelers speed down the highway, the second or third or fourth following way too closely for my comfort as they are sucked along, "drafting" off the truck in front of them.

Many medical groups, especially in hospital-based specialties such as anesthesiology and radiology, appear to be in the process of being sucked down the road to being acquired.

I'm not saying that, for some groups, selling out isn't a perfectly viable plan or, that for other groups, acquiring another group isn't the best strategy.

Rather, I'm saying that you shouldn't be blinded by the meme of the moment, the acquisition meme.

Consider all of your options. Develop your strategy. Groom your group for the intended outcome. Have alternatives. Then launch your tactics.

Don't simply get sucked into something.

I SEE ZOMBIES EVERY DAY

I don't get the zombie thing on TV commercials. But I see zombies every day.

We had to sit in class for most of the day when I was in elementary school. Sitting still was apparently the lesson plan. It sure wasn't the school work.

Perhaps that's why so many people look to others to be told what to do. Or they think someone is actually looking out for them. They're still children, socially and economically. Take care of me, please. I deserve it. It takes a village and that village is going to take care of me. No, it's not.

This isn't just limited to those working unionized factory jobs. "You can't fire me because I'm protected." The reality is that you're trapped by two masters, the employer and the union, and neither wants you to really succeed. The employer wants you to work. The union wants you to pay dues. Both want you to do as you are told. Johnny, don't fidget. Sit still.

Today more physicians than ever before are opting for factory work. Employment by hospitals. It's easy. Less paperwork (really?). It's safe. Until you are laid off. Until you are fired. Until you are subjected to medical staff discipline because you don't follow orders.

The kind of zombies I see are real. They eat human flesh. They consume their own lives, their future, and those dependent upon them.

FROM THE VIRUS' POINT OF VIEW

Fighting viruses blinds you to their point of view. Get inside and replicate.

That's how groups often lose their contracts. A member of the group becomes disgruntled. He stages a revolt. He is now in charge of the group with the contract.

This isn't about how to block that virus. That's another topic.

Instead, think about how physicians should replicate the virus on a larger scale.

Hospitals are busy "aligning" physicians.

Why not take control of the hospital?

Congress has legislated away new physician majority owned hospitals from Medicare participation. It didn't legislate away control.

And just as easily as Congress legislated out physician owned hospitals it can legislate in that hospitals must be controlled by physicians.

Impossible!

If you think it is impossible then it is. But if you think like that microscopic virus that destroyed the patient's body, it's not.

THE ODDS OF MEDICAL GROUP SURVIVAL

My dog stood body frozen stiff yet ready to lunge. His eyes fixed on the only object in his world, the squirrel eating seeds off the ground 14 feet away.

The squirrel matched the stare, glanced at the tree about four feet distant and then, continuing to eat the entire time, just turned his back as if he were the only one who would be doing any eating that day.

Businesses, including medical groups, do the equivalent. In a complex system there are who-knows-how-many unseen risks. But there are many significant, obvious risks as well, risks that may be acknowledged intellectually but ignored as unimportant either because the observer is lying to himself or is unprepared to deal with them.

The squirrel's bet was a good one. My dog's never caught one. But maybe one day he will. For the squirrel it will be low odds times high potential damage (death) equals high risk, ignored.

But it's not that the risk wasn't there every time. It was; it's just that the odds came out in the squirrel's favor that day. For the squirrel in the yard, the odds of being eaten had come out in his favor his entire life.

Medical groups that have had successful 20 or 30 or even longer runs have benefited from a similar run of the dice.

Several years ago, I had another dog, Showlow. I had the task of removing squirrel parts from the back yard on a regular basis, even once having to tell her to drop the head as if we were playing the Addams Family version of fetch.

Value

WHAT A 57 YEAR OLD BURGER JOINT CAN TEACH YOU ABOUT DELIVERING VALUE

During junior high school summers, my friend Steve Cunningham and I would ride our bikes across the San Fernando Valley to buy a root beer (and sometimes a chili cheese burger) at The Munch Box. The root beer was ice cold. The burger hot, it's cheese melty. It was a special blend of distant, delicious, almost forbidden fruit.

I've often recommended that groups provide an Experience Monopoly™ to their customers: an experience for patients, referral sources and facilities that they cannot get from anyone else.

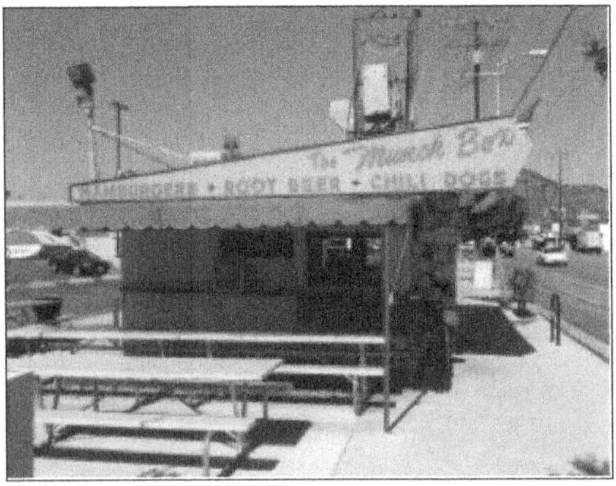

But simply providing an experience isn't enough. At its core, a successful exchange involves delivering value as well.

That's far more complex than it initially appears.

Equal value doesn't cut it. The key is delivering more value than the recipient parts with in return.

The scales balance, but not from some objective point of view, only from a subjective one: from the recipient's perspective.

And strangely, the balance isn't perfectly even. From the recipient's his point of view, it's always tipped in his favor. (But just as magically, the party delivering the value sees an increase in his value as well.)

A dollar for a dollar's worth of value is common, but it will never delight, it will never draw the customer back to you, it will never bind the customer to you.

In creating an Experience Monopoly™ and in delivering value, the key is to metaphorically deliver two dollars for every dollar received. Even better, it's to create a situation in which the recipient interprets the relationship as receiving the two dollars up front, so to speak, even before he or she parts with one.

In an Experience Monopoly™ there's an element of the fear of loss: The customer knows that he or she can't receive the same value from another source. That's extremely important. But there's something else at play, too, something more than fear: That's the pleasure of gain. If I can get two dollars of perceived value from you for every dollar I give you, I'd take my fill every day.

Of course, this begs the question of how you demonstrate value. But's that's another story.

Think of the value Steve and I found at The Munch Box: We rode our bikes a bit more than 9 miles through the 100-plus degree heat and then paid the price in dollars for the root beer and cheeseburger. And we did it time and again.

And even with dozens of fast food places a few minutes away, The Munch Box is still there. Get the idea? (Photo credit: Chester Paul Sgroi)

EFFORTS DON'T NECESSARILY EQUAL VALUE

I recently heard a news story announcing that General Motors was, per its agreement with the Auto Workers Union, making bonus distributions of, as I recall, $8,300 per worker.

Asked to comment, the union spokesperson said that although the workers appreciated the bonus money, it did make up for the fact that they had not received wage hikes for several years.

Completely missing from her comments, and probably from her mind, was the fact that it's only because of a bailout with our money do any of those union members still have jobs at General Motors.

There is a major disconnect here between efforts and the creation of value. This disease doesn't afflict only those working on the manufacturing line at General Motors, but those in the corporate office as well. All of their previous efforts, and I have no reason to doubt that they devoted huge amounts of time and effort to their tasks, resulted in an overall loss of value: cars that didn't sell and costs that ate the company alive.

Value, on the other hand, is determined by the customer.

Of course, this holds true in all areas (excepting those in which the government has meddled, causing more harm than good, say, as in public schools) including healthcare.

Many physician group members, from leaders to newly hired employees, think that merely showing up and doing their cases is what creates value in terms of the ongoing relationship with their facility. It doesn't.

Look, I'm not saying that treating patients isn't of value. What I am saying is that those efforts are not equivalent to the creation of value in terms of the relationship with facilities. The same holds true in connection with the creation of value as to the relationship with referral sources.

One thing's for certain, the government's not going to bail out your medical group.

THIS IS WHAT COMMODITIZED HEALTHCARE LOOKS LIKE

I recently received a box of books from someone I know…well, let me restate that: I received the box minus 2/3 of the books. It seems as if the post office destroyed the box but, instead of putting the rest of the books back in, simply taped the heck out of the box and just kept the rest of the books. Perhaps putting books back in a destroyed box is not part of the job description, while taping up the box is.

It occurred to me that this is a graphic illustration of what commodity healthcare looks like. "We delivered the box. What are you complaining about?!!"

There's no need to show you a picture of a FedEx box. The chances that it would be damaged are almost nil. If it were damaged, the driver would repackage it and make sure it got to you.

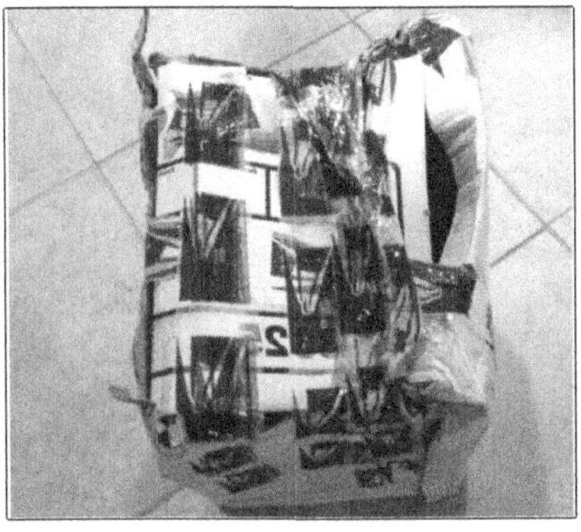

Some people are willing to pay a huge dollar premium to ship FedEx.

Soon, some people will be willing to pay a huge dollar premium to receive non-commodity healthcare.

If you simply want to tape 'em up, then the payoff will be at the commodity level. On the other hand, if you're interested in providing an Experience Monopoly™ to your patients, and in being paid accordingly, this is the time to seriously strategize for that future.

Knowledge Products

BREAKING NEWS ON KICKBACKS: THE LATEST ON THE COMPANY MODEL

The recording of Mark F. Weiss' webinar Breaking News On Kickbacks: The Latest On The Company Model. As the healthcare economy becomes more strained, the pace of illegal kickback activity has increased. Join Mark F. Weiss, attorney for the Requestor of OIG Advisory Opinion 13-15, to learn the absolute latest on the so-called Company Model.

Audio Version $279
Video Version $379
Audio and Video Version $379

To purchase Breaking News On Kickbacks: The Latest On The Company Model go to www.advisorylawgroup.com/knowledgeproducts.html

---

DOUBLE INDEMNITY: PUTTING YOURSELF AT RISK FOR MILLIONS – THE INTERPLAY BETWEEN INSURANCE AND INDEMNIFICATION PROVISIONS IN YOUR HOSPITAL AND PHYSICIAN CONTRACTS

They may look like boilerplate, but your feet might be in the boiler's fire if you haven't properly thought through the impact and interplay of the indemnification and insurance provisions in your contracts with hospitals and with providers.

Audio Version $129
Video Version $179
Video and Audio Versions $179

To purchase **Double Indemnity: Putting Yourself At Risk For Millions – The Interplay Between Insurance And Indemnification Provisions In Your Hospital And Physician Contracts** go to www.advisorylawgroup.com/knowledgeproducts.html

DISRUPTIVE STRATEGIES IN HEALTHCARE: DESIGNING THEM AND DEALING WITH THEM

Believing that the future of the business of healthcare will be a projection of, or incremental improvement over, today's reality is a fool's game.

Although predicting the specifics of the future is impossible, it's certain to involve disruptive strategies. Think, for example, of the disruption to the private practice of medicine resulting from the blossoming hospital-centric worldview. But are you aware of the disruptive strategies aimed at shattering that worldview?

There are only two sides to the healthcare coin: figure out a way to disrupt the current practice model or figure out how to deal with someone else's disruption.

By purchasing you'll understand the role of disruption in healthcare, you'll learn of disruptive events currently on the horizon, you'll learn key elements in designing disruptive strategies and you'll understand how best to protect your practice from someone else's disruption.

Audio Version $107
Video Version $197
Audio and Video Version $197

To purchase **Disruptive Strategies In Healthcare: Designing Them And Dealing With Them**
go to www.advisorylawgroup.com/knowledgeproducts.html

THE FAST™ GROUP--MEDICAL GROUP GOVERNANCE FOR TODAY'S MARKET.

Does Your Group Suffer From This Governance Defect?

"I'll have to get back to you on that, our board doesn't meet until next Saturday."

In an increasingly competitive, increasingly hospital-centric world, the saying "money likes speed" is more true than ever. Yet many medical groups have doomed themselves to stasis, or worse, as a result of their defective governance structure.

Audio Version $97
Video Version $129
Audio and Video Version $129

To purchase **The Fast™ Group--Medical Group Governance For Today's Market.**
go to www.advisorylawgroup.com/knowledgeproducts.html

WHY YOUR MEDICAL GROUP NEEDS A NEW CONTRACTING STRATEGY

No matter your political bent, there's no doubt that society is becoming increasingly affected by "we" think, from concepts of shared sacrifice, to paying your fair share, to "giving back."

These notions of community and cooperation present an advantage to local medical groups in fighting off the onslaught of outside competitors.

But that advantage will be lost unless medical groups adopt a contracting strategy that harmonizes with the growing societal trends.

When you watch or listen to this thirty-minute webinar, you'll learn:

- The major general societal trends.
- How those trends impact medical group relationships.
- How those trends impact medical group facility contracting.
- Why having a strategy that ties into those trends provides you with an essential advantage.

Audio Version $97
Video Version $129
Video and Audio Versions $129

To purchase **Why Your Medical Group Needs A New Contracting Strategy**
go to www.advisorylawgroup.com/knowledgeproducts.html

REVERSE ENGINEERING A NATIONAL TAKEOVER OF YOUR FACILITY CONTRACT

Like a neutron bomb, national or large regional groups wants to take over your facility contract, vaporize your group, and cherry-pick your desirable assets: your physicians and other providers.

By understanding their approach, you'll drastically increase your group's chances for survival.

In the approximately 45 minutes of this recording of an ALG Webinar, you'll learn:

The strategies and tactics national groups use to approach hospitals.
What they are saying about you.
What you can do proactively to inoculate your group against their approach.
Other tools for protecting your group from planned contractual annihilation.

Audio recording: $397
Complete video of webinar: $497
Audio recording and complete video: $497

To purchase **Reverse Engineering A National Takeover Of Your Facility Contract**
go to www.advisorylawgroup.com/knowledgeproducts.html

HOW TO DEAL WITH RFPS FOR PHYSICIAN SERVICES

More and more hospitals are disrupting their relationships with hospital-based and office-based physicians.

The favored tool? The request for proposal, commonly known as an "RFP."

How can an RFP be avoided?

Do you respond?

How do you respond?

How can the rules be bent?

These are among the issues discussed in this recording of an ALG Webinar. You'll receive practical and actionable information for your group's immediate application.

After viewing the recording or listening to the audio of this ALG Webinar, you'll have:

- An understanding of the three types of RFPs
- Knowledge of the strategies and tactics used to avoid RFPs
- Awareness of the major defect in the RFP process
- Knowledge of strategies and tactics used to respond to RFPs
- An understanding of the importance of a strategy aimed outside of the RFP process itself

Purchase How to Deal with RFPs for Physician Services now:

Audio recording: $207
Complete video of webinar: $297
Audio recording and complete video: $297

To purchase **How to Deal With RFPs For Physician Services** go to www.advisorylawgroup.com/knowledgeproducts.html

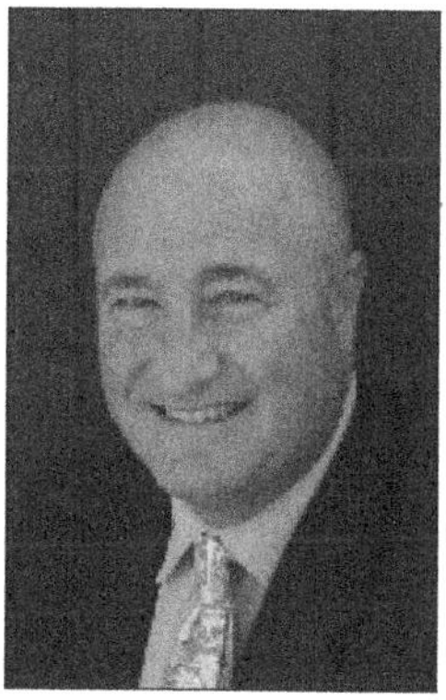

Mark F. Weiss is an expert on the legal and business issues affecting medical groups, entrepreneurial physicians, and healthcare businesses.

Mr. Weiss advises clients nationally on achieving their goals, maximizing their profits and managing their risk of loss.

Lawyers often view the world though a microscope trained to see the minutia of the "legal" issue and, as a result, ignore virtually everything else. As a result, they preach a purely "legal solution" that, quite often, is worthless in terms of any practical benefit for you.

Mr. Weiss views the world differently: He and his firm, The Mark F. Weiss Law Firm, operate on the same entrepreneurial level as do you. He understands that legal issues are intertwined with your business issues and cannot be separated. He understands that psychological and political issues often transcend the obvious issues.

Mr. Weiss is a frequent speaker and the author of more than 200 articles on issues affecting healthcare providers. From 2002 through 2013, he held an appointment as clinical assistant professor of USC's Keck School of Medicine.

Contact Mr. Weiss by email at markweiss@advisorylawgroup.com or by phone at 310.843.2800.